DR. RICHARD E. BUSCH III

*Surgery
not
Included

THE ULTIMATE PUBLISHING HOUSE (TUPH)
49540 – 80 GLEN SHIELDS AVENUE, TORONTO, ONTARIO
CANADA, L4K 2B0

Telephone: 647-883-1758 Fax: 416-228-2598
*www.ultimatepublishinghouse.com*
E-mail: Info@UltimatePublishingHouse.com

US OFFICE:
The Ultimate Publishing House (TUPH)
P.O. Box 1204
Cypress, Texas, U.S.A. 77410
Ordering Information

*Quantity Sales:*
COMPANIES, ORGANIZATIONS, INSTITUTIONS, AND INDUSTRY

PUBLICATIONS:
Quantity discounts are available on bulk purchases of this book for reselling, educational purposes, subscription incentives, gifts, sponsorship, or fundraising. Unique books or book excerpts can also be fashioned to suit specific needs such as private labelling with your logo on the cover and a message from or a message printed on the second page of the book. For more information please contact our Special Sales Department at The Ultimate Publishing House.

Orders for college textbook / course adoption use.
Please contact the Ultimate Publishing House Tel: 647-883-1758

**TUPH** is a registered trademark of The Ultimate Publishing House

PRINTED IN CANADA.
*Surgery not Included by Dr. Richard E. Busch III*

ISBN: 978-0-9819398-4-1

*First Edition*

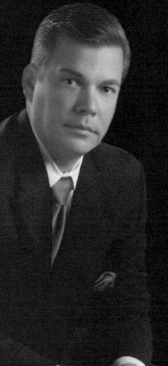

# DR. RICHARD E. BUSCH III

FOREWORD BY LES BROWN,
*International Speaker & Best Selling Author*

\*Surgery
not
Included

# FREEDOM
## from Chronic Neck and Back Pain

# DISCLAIMER

*Surgery not Included™* is not intended to diagnose or prescribe any treatment for any medical or psychological condition(s), nor are there any claims or offers to prevent, diagnose, treat, mitigate, or cure any medical or psychological conditions.

The book contains the ideas and opinions of its author and is intended solely to provide helpful information.

It is offered with the understanding that the author and publisher are not engaged in rendering medical, health or any other kind of personal professional services in the book.

The reader should consult his or her medical, health or other competent professional before adopting any of the suggestions in the book.

The author and publisher specifically disclaim all responsibility for any liability, loss, or risk, personal or otherwise, that is incurred as a consequence (directly or indirectly) of the use and application of any of the contents of this book.

*The book contains the following disclaimer:*
The names of people mentioned in the case studies published within the book have been changed to protect the patient's identities.

# ACKNOWLEDGEMENTS

I would like to thank the following individuals and companies who helped bring this book into being, and thank you to those who encouraged me along the path toward helping patients recover without the need for surgery:

*Dr. and Mrs. Richard E. Busch, Jr.*

*Dr. John R. Ashton*

*Jack Mochamer, Attorney at Law*

*Jaclyn Touzard, Editor of* The American Chiropractor *magazine*

*Elaine Fortmeyer*

*Dee Cee Laboratories®*

*Douglas Laboratories®*

*Enzyme Formulations®*

The American Chiropractor *magazine*

*The Ultimate Publishing House (TUPH) particularly Felicia and Dee*

*I would also like to extend a heartfelt thanks to my wonderful staff and my patients, past, present and future.*

# DEDICATION

**\*Surgery not Included** *is dedicated to my family:*
*Jennifer, my beautiful wife, and*
*Elaina and Olivia, my daughters.*

# FOREWORD

## *Foreword by Les Brown*

Les Brown, founder of Les Brown Enterprises, is the leading authority on releasing human potential and enhancing lives. As a renowned professional speaker, personal development coach, author and former television personality, Les Brown has risen to national and international prominence by capturing audiences with electrifying speeches, challenging them to live up to their greatness. "One of the most important things I've done in my life was to shake off mediocrity and continuously strive to live up to my potential greatness. " In my profession I am very fortunate to meet and have a relationship with other professionals who are at the top of their industry and have lived up to their potential greatness. One such professional is Dr. Richard Busch who has dedicated his life to helping the sick and suffering.

Applied knowledge is power. Because of the devastating impact that disease and sickness can bring into one's life, coupled with the astronomical cost of healthcare, people everywhere are seeking knowledge that can give them the power to improve and maintain optimal health and well-being.

Unfortunately, we live in a society where the response to illness in many cases, is to drug it out, burn it out or cut it out. In this groundbreaking book, *Surgery not Included,* compassionate doctor, dynamic speaker and insightful author Dr. Rick Busch addresses the agonizing and excruciating non-specific back and neck pain that affects millions of people.

*Surgery not Included* takes the reader on an all too familiar journey through the medical merry-go-round that includes endless testing, misdiagnosis and in most cases, ineffective and unnecessary surgery. Committed to stopping this profit-driven, avoidable cycle of pain, drugs and surgery, and in order provide hope for a better and more fulfilled life, Dr. Busch presents a cutting-edge integrated medical approach that will empower you in order to provide hope, to take control of your health.

The most compelling aspect of this book is Dr. Busch's focus on the whole patient. I've often said, "If you do not feel well, you can not do well." Dr. Busch understands that back or neck pain affects not just your body but every aspect of your existence, including your job, your relationships and your quality of life. Understanding that pain is emotional and psychological, as well as physical, Dr. Busch seeks to heal his patients from the inside out.

Many people are convinced that their only choices are to live with chronic back pain or undergo invasive surgery and prolonged recovery. The idea that pain can be healed in a few short weeks with very little downtime seems too good to be true – but it is true. With more than a decade of experience combining the ideas of holistic health with technological advancements in the field of non-surgical pain relief, Dr. Busch has helped thousands of patients reclaim their lives – without surgery. In this eye-opening book, he uses real-life examples to illustrate the healing of patients from a variety of situations and with a various medical conditions.

It is very difficult to write for both patients and doctors. Dr. Busch has found that fine line. He not only writes in a style that will intrigue doctors, but through the use of simple language and diagrams, he allows the layperson to grasp the concepts as well.

As stated earlier, applied knowledge is power. While the information that Dr. Busch provides is invaluable, he also advises that patients must apply that knowledge by taking responsibility for their own healthcare. They cannot expect healthcare professionals always to think of their best interests. Dr. Busch arms people with the tools and knowledge to be an informed participant in their own recovery, letting them know they are not trapped between their pain and surgery. The most important message you can gain out of this book is that you have options, there is a better way but you must take action.

Underlying the medical information and practical advice, in this book is a road map that will give you the insight needed to reclaim your health and live a life of love, happiness and comfort. Well done Dr. Busch - *Surgery not Included.

**Les Brown,** *Les Brown Enterprises*

# CONTENTS

# CHAPTER 1

*Back Pain is Universal*

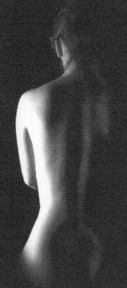

# CHAPTER ONE

*Back Pain is Universal*

The American Chiropractic Association estimates that as many as 80% of Americans will experience back pain at some time in their lives, and as many as 31 million are experiencing back pain at any one time. The numbers may seem astronomical, but the latest numbers from the Bureau of Labor Statistics report that back pain is responsible for 62% of people who miss work. None of us has to look too far to find real life examples of people with back or neck problems, and many of us have had personal experience.

## Cumulative Pain

IF YOU ARE over the age of 40, the likelihood that you will experience episodes of back pain is increasingly prevalent. You may have had a back or neck injury years or even decades ago, and at that time, it appeared to be asymptomatic or resolved. However, the condition may be cumulative as the damage to soft tissue and bone results in continuing degeneration, and the result is back or neck pain that can appear later in life.

This can be confusing, since a recent onset of pain may appear to have started from something as ordinary as stepping off a curb, sleeping in an awkward position, or playing a weekend game of touch football. This episode of pain is acute and sudden, but the underlying cause can be linked to the original injury or condition. Minor, intermittent episodes of pain have likely been occurring all along, yet they are not thought of as a chronic, ongoing condition, or related to the original injury.

## *Pain Does Not Warrant Care*

MANY PEOPLE LIVE with chronic or ongoing pain because they do not perceive their pain to be severe enough to warrant care. What they do not realize is that because the conditions causing back or neck pain are cumulative, much more long-term damage may be incurred by not addressing their current symptoms. While the original injury may have seemed insignificant, the body compensates. Function is limited and continues to cause damage at the site of the injury. Many times, a disc condition may result.

How many family members and colleagues do you know who have had painful flare-ups years later that they credited to an "old football injury"? A chronic neck or back condition can develop years after a motor vehicle accident. In the meantime, the old injury may have been repeatedly aggravated, and the degenerative process just keeps getting worse. Eventually, the cumulative cycle escalates to the point where it results in a disc-related condition, and the sufferer can no longer work and function normally.

It is common for pain sufferers to be unaware of the progression of their pain. Social or cultural attitudes and conditioning may cause people to deny or even hide their pain. An example of pain progression would be increased tingling or discomfort, or numbness, in the arms or legs. Living with a level of discomfort becomes "normal," and it may take a major increase in intensity or frequency of pain— changing from inconvenient pain to a loss of function, or from intermittent to constant pain—to cause someone to seek treatment.

Since back and neck pain are subjective, many people who suffer will self diagnose and self-medicate with over-the-counter (OTC) pain relievers that may help for a short time.

While OTC products may be generally safe and non-addictive, they do pose risks when taken incorrectly or over long periods. All medications have side effects, even OTC products. Eventually the sufferer must talk to a doctor or make lifestyle modifications.

## *Problems with the Diagnosis*

THE ORIGIN OF back and neck pain can be nonspecific. The spine is complex—composed of bones, nerves, ligaments, muscles, and cartilage—so the condition causing the pain can be difficult to pinpoint. A condition can create numerous symptoms and have the potential for a multitude of possible diagnoses. Often, it can be difficult for a patient to get a definitive diagnosis from the doctor about the source of pain.

In addition, there are varying terms or descriptions regarding spinal conditions, and there is a lack of uniformity among doctors when using medical terminology. Some terms that patients may hear from different doctors for the same condition are pinched nerve, bulging disc, slipped disc, herniated disc, and ruptured disc. It is no wonder that a patient can be confused about a diagnosis and uncertain of the best treatment option.

As a chiropractor, I diagnose and treat patients who have chronic pain and severe disc conditions, such as herniated disc and degenerative disc disease, and their pain is interfering with their normal daily activities.

George, a 32-year-old construction worker, is an example of a patient who had chronic pain due to lumbar degenerative disc disease. George started having low back problems when he was 10. He was a typical kid who fell out of trees, fell off his bike, and played contact sports. All the injuries led to cumulative back problems that needed to be addressed and were causing problems later in his life. Throughout his adult life, he suffered from bouts of intermittent low back pain that he ignored the majority of the time, and he treated it with OTC products.

Periodically, when George's pain was severe enough, he sought chiropractic care, and it helped temporarily. However, he never achieved long-term relief because he never continued with the care. Then one day, when he was working at a construction site, he tried to lift a wooden-framed wall, and he was immobilized by excruciating leg and back pain.

For five long weeks, George suffered miserably, and he took large doses of OTC remedies. Finally, his wife, fed up with seeing him suffer, called a chiropractor. After three treatments, George was significantly worse. He was incapacitated. He could not even get out of bed to get to the bathroom.

When George's wife called my office, I recommended that they immediately call an ambulance and take him to an emergency room.

At the hospital, George was sedated to enable the staff to perform an MRI. The hospital admitted George, and he was heavily medicated. He stayed for two days. His diagnosis was torn hip ligaments and two herniated lumbar discs. The doctors told George that lumbar surgery was inevitable, but he refused because he had not been able to work for more than six weeks, and he could not tolerate months of recovery, physical therapy, and the loss of income.

The hospital released George, and he came to me for an evaluation. After an examination and review of the MRI films, I was confident George was a solid candidate for treatment with the nonsurgical DRS Protocol™. Within two days of beginning care, his pain had decreased significantly, and he was moving around without help. Within five weeks, George was back to work. Within eight weeks, he had 100% resolution of pain. *Surgery not Included.

Many people are fearful of surgery, and with good reason. A multitude of unknowns can occur when we choose to move forward with a surgical procedure. There are potential risks from anesthesia and scar tissue. Additionally, the potential for fracture, coma, paralysis, permanent nerve damage, and damage to the vertebrae exists, along with bleeding and clotting complications (that may be life threatening or may require transfusion), plus the MRSA bacteria and other contagious infections (that may require additional surgery). Certain preexisting diseases and medical conditions—including diabetes, malnutrition, obesity, smoking, alcoholism, substance abuse, immune and connective tissue diseases, heart disease, kidney disease, cancer, depression, and high blood pressure—will increase the potential for failed surgery outcomes and complications. A critical concern is that no one can guarantee a successful outcome from spinal surgery. Of course, there is always the possibility of death when patients undergo anesthesia.

Many patients I treat have had one or more failed back or neck surgeries. They did not have pain relief, and in some cases, surgery made their conditions worse. A notable number of these patients have had revision surgeries, which have an even higher risk of failure, and the likelihood of failure increases with each subsequent surgery.

Surgical outcomes are uncertain because the spine is complex. Surgery is a risky proposition because of the inherent risks of an operation and complicating factors from preexisting medical conditions. In addition, there is risk because of the close proximity of the discs to the spinal cord. Residual effects can be scar tissue and nerve damage. It is for these reasons that no one can guarantee you will be pain-free or even experience significant long-term improvement from back or neck surgery.

At specific times, surgery is indicated, and for some patients surgery can be successful. For others, it can have serious consequences and complications. Surgery should be the absolute last option. Once surgery is performed, it cannot be undone.

Some additional residual effects of surgery can be as follows: numbness, tingling, change of gait due to muscle weakness, change of flexibility of the spine, and accelerated degeneration, even when the procedure is considered a success. Unless you have an emergency condition, it should be imperative that you explore every possible treatment option to avoid surgery for a spinal disc condition, and to allow your body to heal through noninvasive treatment methods such as the DRS Protocol™.

# *The Spine*

OFTEN, PEOPLE DO not give serious thought to their spine, even though it provides numerous vital functions. The spine allows humans to stand in an upright position and gives the body a supportive framework. One of its essential functions is to house and protect the spinal cord and nerve roots, which allow the brain to send and receive signals from all parts of the body, including the internal organs. The spine also provides flexibility. It is where muscles, ligaments, and tendons attach to anchor the arms and legs. This provides the ability to walk, stand, and hold the head upright.

The spinal column is composed of 24 stacked vertebrae, or bone. Between each vertebra is a soft disc that acts like a small gel pillow, or a jelly doughnut. The discs function as shock absorbers that stop the vertebrae from bumping and rubbing against each other. When you jump, fall, or walk, the discs absorb the shock and vibration, and they keep the vertebrae from jarring and causing damage to each other and your nervous system.

Ligaments, an essential part of the skeletal system, are strong, rubbery bands of connective tissue that hold the joints, bones, cartilage, and skeletal structures together and hold the discs in place. Ligaments flex, which allows bones their necessary movement but still enables them to maintain the structure of the skeleton.

Tendons are fibrous, inelastic bands of tissue that attach muscles to the bone. The spine also has joints, called facet joints, which link and stabilize the vertebrae and allow them to move much like a knee or elbow.

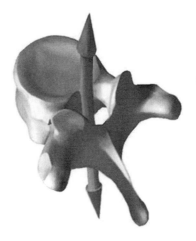

**Spinal Canal**
The arrow
illustrates
the hole in the
vertebra or the
intervertebral
canal

AS SHOWN IN the preceding illustration, each vertebra has a hole in the center, called the intervertebral canal, that houses and protects the spinal cord. The spinal cord, a bundle of nerve fibers, is surrounded by tissue and fluid, and is protected by vertebrae. On each side of the spinal column, nerve bundles branch out in pairs of spinal nerves. Because of these nerves, a spinal injury can easily cause pain.

When a doctor discusses back or neck pain, he or she will refer to four main spinal regions. One region is the cervical spine, consisting of seven vertebrae, which begins at the base of the skull and continues to the base of the neck. The adjacent region, the thoracic spine, consisting of 12 vertebrae, begins at the top of the shoulders and goes to the bottom of the rib cage. The next area is the lumbar spine, generally consisting of five vertebrae. Below that is the sacrum, more commonly referred to as the tailbone, which connects the spine to the pelvis.

Muscles are composed of both cells and fiber. The muscles next to the spine are the paraspinal muscles, and these run lengthwise along the spine. They attach to the vertebrae and support the spine. There are two layers of muscle. One lies on top of the other. These muscles, when injured and strained, go into spasm to decrease movement, even if the injury is in another part of the spine.

When you understand how many structures the spine protects and the multiple functions it performs, it is easy to recognize the potential for frequent injury. Injuries can be due to accidents, overuse, abuse, and pushing the spine beyond its natural limits. The result is pain.

## *From Pain, Diagnosis to Disappointment*

PAIN IS OUR body's alarm system. It causes a protective reflex, and in the case of back or neck injury, pain may initiate "muscle guarding" in order to avoid further tissue or nerve damage. Pain will persist because of inflammation and irritation of the nerves.

Pain is a unique and personal experience. You cannot see the pain, you cannot smell the pain, and you cannot touch the pain. Pain can only be ranked by the patient reporting the pain on a scale. The scale ranges from zero to ten—zero signifies the absence of pain and ten is unbearable pain. You cannot see pain on an X-ray or through other diagnostic tests. Pain is not measured like weight or blood pressure. Although X-rays, blood samples, and other tests can detect problems that might cause it, pain cannot be seen.

Many times, when a patient is seen by a doctor for back or neck pain, the doctor will address only the complaints the patient verbalizes and not proceed further than medicating the symptoms.

Everyone experiences pain differently. How the brain interprets pain is subjective, and it is influenced by a multitude of emotional and physical factors, such as the sufferer's personality, underlying health conditions, along with physical and genetic makeup, previous episodes of pain, preconceived ideas about pain, and the influence of drugs, whether prescription or recreational.

Because the causes of back and neck pain can be complex, in some cases self-limiting or short-term, physicians are often reluctant to invest too much time into determining the source of the pain, and they often do not find anything specific in the initial examination. The diagnosis will likely be "nonspecific" pain.

If an initial diagnosis, such as nonspecific back pain, is given on the first visit, this may impede further diagnosing that could have been made through imaging or other diagnostic testing, unless the patient continues to complain. There are standard guidelines for medical doctors, published in the October 2007 issue of *Annals of Internal Medicine,* that recommend they categorize patients with back pain into three general categories: nonspecific low back pain, back pain that may be associated with spinal conditions, and back pain that may be associated with other causes, such as cancer. The majority of patients—85%—fall into the first category. The guidelines further recommend that doctors should not order imaging or other diagnostic tests such as MRIs or X-rays for nonspecific back pain patients. The guidelines recommend that those tests should be reserved for patients suspected of having more serious underlying conditions, such as infection or cancer. Paraphrasing a past president of the American Pain Society, the mystery begins with the first visit to the doctor and then continues from there, since the exact cause of back pain is never found in 85% of patients.

Developing an accurate diagnosis for neck and back pain can be significantly more difficult than for other medical conditions. The diagnoses of some conditions, such as fractures, tumors, and pathology, are clear. However, many musculoskeletal conditions, which have to do with muscles, bones, tendons, ligaments, joints, and cartilage, are considerably more difficult to diagnose.

## The Disappointed Patient

IT CAN BE difficult for a patient who has already seen a doctor, followed the recommended course of treatment while being disappointed with the results, and perhaps even have been dismissed or put off by a doctor, to have the heart to listen to yet another doctor who supposedly has the answer. I have treated numerous patients who took a long time and went through much uncertainty before finally deciding to come to me for treatment. One of the most memorable was Wes, a 40-year-old engineer.

Fifteen years before I saw Wes, he fell 25 feet down a manhole and seriously injured his back. Years later, he was still in significant pain, but his neurologist said there was no identifiable reason he should have any pain. Another specialist told him he had eight bulging discs, and he needed surgery. Prior to coming to me for an initial consultation, Wes had been treated with three to four epidural injections a year since the time of his accident. After evaluating Wes, I was absolutely convinced I could help him by using the DRS Protocol™. However, Wes had lived with his pain for so long, and had been injected with so many epidurals that did not help, that the idea of a comfortable, easy, and pain-free treatment seemed too good to be true. Because of his treatment history, he was understandably skeptical of my recommendations. He honestly did not believe there was any procedure or treatment that could eliminate his pain, and that it would be without surgery.

Wes did not begin treatment right away. He continued treatment with a pain specialist, and this consisted of injections in his lower back every three to six months. The pain relief was less effective with each injection. However, not long after my consultation with Wes, his wife came for a consultation and began treatment for a disc condition. Immediately, she had relief from the pain and she was extremely pleased with her results. A brief time later, Wes' mother-in-law started care for degenerative disc disease and she had more than satisfactory results also. It was interesting that Wes would strongly encourage both of these important women in his life to undergo treatment with the DRS Protocol™. Apparently, he was not convinced that I could help him.

Finally, Wes came for treatment, and within a few weeks, he was experiencing tremendous relief. Today, he water skis barefoot and is more active than he would have dared imagine.

It is very important for anyone with a severe disc condition, when given a choice between living with pain or enduring invasive and sometimes risky procedures, to research alternative procedures such as the DRS Protocol™. It is necessary to get a second, nonsurgical opinion. I have helped thousands of patients understand that their lives do not have to remain limited by the painful aftereffects of spinal injuries or disease. Even if patients have had previous back or neck surgeries and still experience pain, they can be helped. Most patients achieve significant changes within a few weeks, and the concept of a noninvasive pain-free treatment, the DRS Protocol™, certainly makes it worth investigating.

Throughout this book, I have included numerous cases from my practice, illustrating a variety and range of symptoms, injuries, and medical issues, to demonstrate that no matter what the situation, there can be hope. Pain need not remain an ever-present reality in your life. The choice to seek nonsurgical and noninvasive treatments is available. It is my hope that many will.

## *Back-and-Neck Pain Pipeline*

ONCE BACK OR neck pain begins to influence the choices of everyday life, the afflicted person normally sees the family doctor for a first level of care. I treat many patients who have followed a similar treatment pattern. I have since labeled this pattern the "back-and-neck pain pipeline." After that has not succeeded in providing relief, many patients come to me to be evaluated for the DRS Protocol™. General practitioners are trained to look for the simplest explanation when confronted with a patient who reports having back pain. In the medical world, it is common to hear the phrase, "If you hear hoof beats, look for horses, not zebras." In other words, they know that minor pain is often caused by temporary inflammation, and it may or may not clear up on its own, so they concentrate on treating the inflammation and pain rather than searching for the underlying source of the pain. This usually results in the patient leaving with prescriptions for muscle relaxants, steroids, or any of a variety of pain medications.

This is merely the first step many patients take in their quest for help and pain relief. They often must convince their doctor that treatments are not working before they are considered to have a serious problem.

The next step of care is often physical therapy (PT). The patient has taken the medications, but they are not working. The doctor then may recommend four to six weeks of physical therapy in an attempt to promote healing, restore function, and just work the problem out. In the case of disc-related back or neck pain, there are two common outcomes of physical therapy: either a patient will have temporary relief, or the pain increases and the patients drops out of therapy. Either way, the patient typically returns to the family doctor's office for the third stage.

At this time, the physician concedes that this is not the average, temporary, weekend-warrior pain, or that the patient is in the nonspecific back pain category. If the symptoms are chronic and severe, then the patient is now in a specialist's territory. The general practitioner then refers the patient to a specialist, likely an orthopedic surgeon or a neurologist. The specialist will test, identify, and treat (it is hoped) the real cause of the pain. Since the obvious diagnoses—nonspecific back pain, strain or sprain—have already been eliminated, the specialist orders diagnostic imaging, which could include X-rays or magnetic resonance imaging (MRI). X-rays are useful in viewing skeletal structure and detecting breaks, bone disease, biomechanical alterations, and degenerative conditions. An MRI creates a magnetic field around the body, sends radio waves though the body to detect changes in molecules, and creates pictorial slices of the body. An MRI is beneficial for viewing soft tissue such as nerves, muscles, ligaments, and organs, as well as bones. Both X-rays and MRIs are excellent tools for seeing the placement and alignment of the spine as well as the damage to the surrounding tissue. Another tool is the CAT scan (computerized axial tomography) or CT scan, which uses X-rays to create a comprehensive, computerized X-ray scan of an area rather than individual images.

Other diagnostic tests include electromyography, or EMG. Needles are inserted directly into the muscles to test the electrical function of the muscles. Another test is nerve conduction velocity, or NCV. During this test, electrodes are taped to the skin, and an uncomfortable shock is experienced. A NCV tests the electrical function of the nerves. The myelogram is a test in which a dye is injected into the spinal column, and it enables the doctor to see, via fluoroscopic X-rays, any bulge within the interveterbral canal that may be putting pressure on the spinal cord or spinal nerves. A discogram is a study in which dye is injected into a specific disc to determine the integrity of the disc itself. A discogram is generally performed to confirm any internal tearing of the annulus (a disc wall). Many of these tests are frequently painful and can be expensive, and they are typically performed in a surgical setting.

A specialist, perhaps an orthopedist, will usually recommend temporarily treating the pain with an epidural injection. Epidurals may help some patients with short-term pain relief and reduction of inflammation. They are performed in a surgical setting, and there may be a series of injections, over time, while the patient continues taking pain medications. Epidurals are injections of medication directly into the epidural space in the spinal column. This is similar to the type of injection many women receive during childbirth. However, the medications injected for back pain are different from those used for childbirth. These injections can be painful and carry risks, including ongoing headaches, nerve damage, and nausea, among other even more serious complications. Research published in the prestigious international medical journal *Spine* (January 1, 2009, Volume 34) indicates that spinal injection therapy used for chronic low back pain has questionable outcomes, and that there is insufficient evidence to support the use of injection therapy because there is a lack of research evidence.

## *Surgical Procedures*

IF THESE TEMPORARY procedures do not work, the usual next step is for the orthopedic surgeon or neurosurgeon to recommend surgery: either a discectomy, in which the discs protruding between the vertebrae are trimmed, or a fusion, in which the vertebrae are stabilized by being fused together using bone graft, metal rods, and screws. Surgery presents a host of risks, and the least serious one on the list is infection and the most severe is permanent disability.

Sometimes a patient is referred to a neurologist. Unfortunately, the conclusion is often the same—a recommendation of surgery—because that is what a surgeon does.

According to *Pathophysiology of Chronic Back Pain* (WebMD, July 9, 2007, by Anthony H. Wheeler, MD, Pain and Orthopedic Neurology), Dr. Wheeler concludes that surgerical procedures for disc-related pain are the most common procedures in the United States, and at a rate that is 40% higher than in any other country.

Surgery will help some cases, although many of these surgeries will have short-term results. Moreover, this may only be the beginning of a patient's journey in attempting to find help.

Periodically, I talk with a physiatrist, a medical doctor who specializes in physical medicine, and we have discussed the long-term outcomes of our patients. He had worked within an orthopedic group for years. During one conversation, he confided that he had left the group after a disagreement on the management of their patients. The majority of their patients who had herniated or degenerative discs were operated on without exploring all of the conservative treatments available, and often, never considering any of them. He told me that, in his professional opinion, the problem was surgery. Surgery may help a percentage of patients for the short-term, but it often creates long-term problems. For that reason, he decided to leave the group. I told him that with my treatment option, the DRS Protocol™, I have had a strong track record, even with patients who have had failed back and neck surgeries. He stopped and said, "Can you just imagine how great your success rates would be if these patients had never been operated on in the first place?"

An article in *Prevention Magazine,* July 2008, entitled "Where You Live Determines Your Quality of Care," notes that the reason why back surgery is recommended may be as simple as the geographical region where the patient lives. Although no one can really know for certain, statistics from Medicare data show there are specific areas in the United States that have considerably higher per capita rates of back surgery than others do. In some areas, the rates are as much as 20% higher. The conclusion is that this could be considered a "surgical signature" or practice style. When the best treatment is unclear, doctors may simply follow the trend in the area.

Surgery may immediately relieve pain, but it is not the lasting solution that many think it is. Surgery can only provide relief if a patient is experiencing pain from direct pressure on a nerve. Surgery does not offer any improvement at all in many cases. There are no guarantees with surgery, and you can never have a surgery undone.

Once these measures are exhausted, patients often still have pain. They are frequently told that the only treatment available to them is to manage their pain through medications, nerve ablation (destroying the nerve), or even spinal cord stimulators. The doctors have exhausted all they know and so they conclude that the patient must find a way to live with the pain. At this point, a patient may be given antidepressants (such as Amitriptyline and Cymbalta®), if the doctor feels the pain might be increasing due to emotional stress or depression, and because these drugs have migrated into chronic pain treatment. In theory, some earlier antidepressants may block the pain pathway.

I successfully treat many patients who have gone through part, or all, of this pain pipeline. Even if patients have had surgery, with limited or no resolution of their problems, they can still experience improvement through the nonsurgical intervention of the DRS Protocol™.

It is estimated that Americans spend more than $50 billion each year on back pain through medication and lost time away from work. The true cost to the patient, besides the loss of income and money spent, is lost time and lost quality of life due to pain, poor outcomes, and the stress placed on him or her and their families.

## *The Real Causes of Back and Neck Pain*

THE CAUSES OF back and neck pain can be narrowed to four major categories. The most common are herniated or bulging discs and degenerative disc disease.

Discs are the soft pads of tissue that fit neatly between each vertebra and act as shock absorbers. These discs separate and protect the bones from clanking together or breaking under stress. A disc is made of a fibrous outer layer, the annulus fibrosis, which surrounds a jelly-like center called the nucleus pulposus. Wear and tear over time, or a sudden fall or other injury, can weaken or tear this outer layer and allow the soft jelly material of the disc to push out, causing a bulge that can press on the surrounding nerves. This is referred to as a bulging or herniated disc, and this causes pain or weakness in the patient.

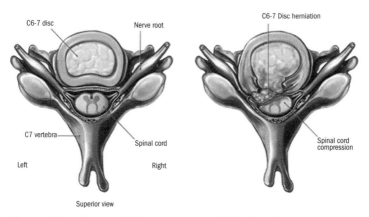

**Normal Vertebra and Disc**          **C6-7 Disc Herniation**

ANOTHER COMMON CAUSE of back and neck pain is degenerative disc disease. As with all parts of the body, the discs of the spine degenerate over time and lose some of their ability to absorb the normal stresses placed on the spine. Because discs are avascular and do not have their own blood supply, they must rely on a process known as diffusion to receive the nutrients, water, and oxygen needed to remain healthy. An impeded blood supply to the spine will reduce the amount of oxygen and nutrients that would normally be supplied to the discs, and the discs go into a state of dehydration or desiccation. This produces a low-grade, chronic inflammation, which causes pressure on the delicate spinal nerves. The area of the body controlled by a compressed nerve will begin to malfunction. This can cause numbness and tingling in the hands or feet, or muscle weakness in the arms or legs. If left untreated, nerve compression can cause substantial and perhaps permanent damage. Degenerative discs also will become much more susceptible to injury from physical stress and even day-to-day activities.

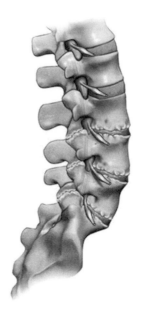

**Degenerative
Discs**
**L3-4**
**L4-5**
**L5-S1**

ANOTHER VERY COMMON pain that is related to herniated or degenerated discs is sciatic pain, which refers to pain along the length of the sciatic nerve, the largest nerve in the body. The sciatic nerve branches off the spine at the pelvis and travels down each leg. A problem at the root of this nerve, where the nerve exits the spine, may be felt along the entire length of the leg and can cause leg weakness. Sciatic pain can be severe and debilitating. Patients often misinterpret this as a problem with their legs, when the primary cause is the result of a bulging disc compressing a nerve at the base of the spine. Sometimes, with severe inflammation, pain will also be felt in the hips and buttocks.

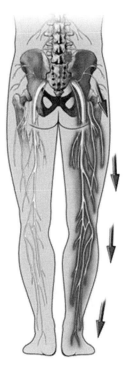

**Sciatic Pain Distribution Pattern**

MANY PEOPLE OVER the age of 50 may experience spinal stenosis, which can be a part of the natural aging process. The spine changes with age and degenerates over time, which can—and will—cause pain. The spine protects the spinal cord by surrounding it with vertebrae and encasing it in spinal fluid. However, when a disc bulges or the soft tissue around the spinal cord becomes inflamed, the soft tissue can push into the spinal canal thereby causing a narrowing, which results in a compression of the spinal cord. Narrowing can also occur in the canals that branch off the spinal cord. While spinal stenosis is most often seen as a condition associated with aging, it can also occur in young people who have had a spinal injury or other abnormal narrowing of the spinal canal. Spinal stenosis is also caused by scar tissue from a previous back or neck surgery. Diseases such as arthritis and scoliosis can cause spinal stenosis as well. It most often occurs in the lumbar spine, but can also occur in the cervical and thoracic spine. When nerves in the lower back (or lumbar spine region) are compressed, they may become inflamed, causing pain in the skin, buttocks, and legs.

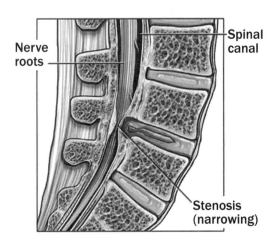

**Spinal Stenosis**

WHEN YOU RUN your hand along your back, you will feel bony protrusions. These are known as spinous processes, and they serve as attachment points for the ligaments and tendons of muscles. Facet joints at each segment of the spine add strength, flexibility, and integrity, as well as offer a range of defined movement (rotation, flexion, and extension) for each vertebral level. Facet joints are similar to other joints in the body, such as the knees and hips.

Facet joints work as a pair in the back of each vertebra. They link the vertebrae above and below, allowing movement of the spine, and are the areas where the vertebrae move and actually touch one another. If the very small amount of tissue between these facet joints, the articular cartilage of the joint capsule, becomes irritated, it can cause the same symptoms that are found with any other pinched nerve: pain, numbness, tingling, and a burning sensation in the lumbar spine. Pain will often show up just in the low back or the buttocks, and this might be referred to as facet syndrome. Facet syndrome in the neck might cause headaches or shoulder pain.

In many cases, when doctors talk about arthritis of the spine, they are referring to the facet joints. These joints cause a patient who has arthritis in the neck to hear grinding when turning the head, due to the rough surfaces of the cartilage rubbing together. This can be disturbing, and not to mention, painful.

*Illustration next page.*

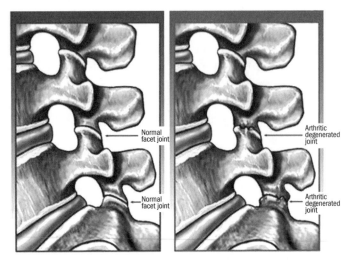

**Normal Facet Joint**          **Arthritic Degenerated Facet Joint**

THERE CAN BE many other causes of back and neck pain, but I have listed the most frequent diagnoses that I treat in my practice. It is interesting that several of these common conditions are associated with age. It is extremely important to understand the cumulative effect that back pain will have in your life, even if you feel that it is "not that bad" right now. I see hundreds of patients every year who have waited until their pain became unbearable. This is completely unnecessary when relief can be easily obtained.

The experience of going through the back-and-neck pain pipeline discourages many who seek relief for their pain but do not want to risk the consequences of surgery. Sometimes it is assumed that the majority of people seeking relief from back or neck pain are older, but this is an invalid assumption. Back pain is the most frequent cause of inactivity in people younger than 45 years old. In fact, I treat children and young people in their teens and twenties.

One such patient is a 16-year-old girl named Lacy. Lacy is a gymnast and cheerleader. One day in cheerleading practice, she landed hard on her backside. She developed back pain and had a hard time doing the normal acrobatic moves she was used to doing. Lacy had some chiropractic care and saw an orthopedist. She was diagnosed with a herniated L5 disc in her lower back. Lacy was treated with rounds of medication and physical therapy and received two epidural injections. The first injection helped for a short time; the second one made her worse. She could not sleep or lay down without discomfort. She was taking large doses of OTC anti-inflammatory medication just to get through the day.

Lacy's doctors told her that the only treatment course for improvement was surgery. However, surgery would have prevented her from participating in her normal activities for an extended period, and there was a high probability that she would never return to all of her previous pursuits.

Lacy's parents decided they wanted nonsurgical intervention before committing their daughter to the surgical path. Once surgery is done, it cannot be undone, and at the age of 16, there is a lifetime of consequences if it does not turn out well. Lacy started treatment immediately, and within a few weeks, her pain had decreased considerably. Within only five weeks, she was back to her normal activity level, and surgery was not necessary. To date, she has had no further problems. The body can heal itself, given the proper environment. *Surgery not Included.

# CHAPTER 2

*The Painful Truth*

# CHAPTER TWO

## *The Painful Truth*

I f you were to walk into a room filled with 100 people and ask how many are suffering or have suffered from back pain, the results might be shocking. Low back pain is the second most common reason for all physician visits in the United States. We also know that 50% of all United States workers admit to having back pain in the last year, and 25% of all adults in America admit to having at least one full day of back pain in the last three months. These are staggering numbers. Of those 100 people, there would be very few who had not experienced some type of back pain.

People often assume that back problems are the result of injury or some underlying chronic disease, such as cancer. This is rarely the case. Most back pain occurs in otherwise healthy people.

A good example of this situation is a patient of mine, a woman named Pat, who was an otherwise very healthy person. Pat awoke one morning with numbness in her right arm. She knew something was seriously wrong and contacted her family doctor. She was given pain medication and told to return if there was no improvement. By the next day, a nerve affecting her arm had become inflamed and she was losing motor function. It was so bad that she could not hold a cup of coffee. By the middle of that night, the pain had intensified to the point that she went to the emergency room, where they administered an injection for the pain.

The next day, Pat had to be driven to her family doctor. The doctor told her that she had two slipped discs and that surgery was her only option. Pat said she felt at that point she was being rushed along an assembly line without knowing all the details, or understanding what was about to happen, or why she had no options other than surgery. She called my office in a panic while still sitting in her family doctor's parking lot. She hoped I could help, and that surgery would not be the inevitable decision. After a thorough evaluation, I determined that she could be helped by my treatment, the DRS Protocol™. Pat's painful ordeal had already caused her to use all her vacation time, and she had to begin short-term disability. Within a few weeks of starting treatment, Pat was able to return to work, and is now free from pain.

I see patients just like Pat every day who desperately hope there is treatment for their pain. I am happy to tell them that there is— *Surgery not Included.

## We Live at Risk

THE LIFESTYLE OF most Americans, as well as most people in the Western world, puts us at increased risk for back pain. Since the majority of back pain is not caused by trauma or disease, what are the real underlying risk factors?

The spine is often perceived to be just a bony structure that is impervious to the factors that affect our overall health, but this is not the reality. The structures of the spine are very sensitive to other health issues and respond to similar risk factors. For example, obesity is reaching epidemic proportions in our country, and the additional pounds affect the spine. This can become apparent in a variety of ways, one of which is determined by where you carry the extra weight. If you carry the weight all in front, as many men do, it can increase the strain on the lower back and pull the vertebrae out of their normal alignment. This biomechanical change can mean that there is increased intradiscal pressure and joint movement, which can cause accelerated degeneration leading to chronic irritation and increased pressure on the nerves. Even if it does not cause pain, the increased pressure on the soft tissue structures (ligaments, discs, and nerves) can lead to the risk of severe injuries from everyday activities.

Poor dietary choices not only may cause obesity, they can also cause deficiencies, imbalances, and inadequate digestion, which are major causes of health problems, including headaches, arthritis, and inflammation. Proper nutrition is imperative for maintaining the health of our bodies, and that includes the discs inside the spinal column. The medical community is acknowledging the connection between chronic diseases and diet:

> *It is becoming increasingly apparent that chronic degenerative diseases (chronic inflammatory states) are evidence of food enzyme deficiency. The 1988 Surgeon General's Report on Health and Nutrition stated unequivocally that chronic degenerative diseases are dietary related.*

*AutoIntoxication* by **Dr. Howard Loomis, Jr.**

One of the most preventable risk factors is smoking. You may think it is ridiculous that smoking can affect the spine, but smoking decreases blood oxygen levels. This means that the discs between the vertebrae of the spine and the nerves are not getting enough oxygen and nutrients to keep them healthy. Not only does this make smokers more vulnerable to injury, smoking also inhibits the healing process and can lead to chronic pain. Smokers are also more prone to disc problems as smoking leaches calcium from connective tissue such as cartilage, ligaments, muscles, and nerves—all of which make up a large part of the spine.

Studies have shown that smoking reduces the blood supply to bones. Nicotine slows the production of bone-forming cells (osteoblasts) and impairs the absorption of calcium. With less bone mineral, smokers develop fragile bones, or osteoporosis.

Being a couch potato can also lead to back pain. If you lead a largely sedentary life, then you are not maintaining strength of the bones and muscles in your back or neck. Studies involving astronauts following space missions show a decrease in weight-bearing activities diminishes bone density and muscle strength. Even if a person has been active, if there has been a significant period of inactivity due to an injury or illness, it is advisable to ease into an exercise regimen. This includes warming up and stretching before activities.

Remember the Victorian-era old movies, in which the grandmother was always harping about good posture? Well, she was right, especially in today's work environment, where employees often stay in one seated position for endless hours. Good posture can prevent a great deal of fatigue and strain on the spine. Poor posture can add strain and stress to the muscles and the spine. The stress of poor posture can change the anatomical structure of the spine over time, which can constrict blood vessels and put pressure on nerves, as well as cause muscle spasms while contributing to disc and joint conditions. Many repetitive stress injuries could be prevented with good posture or the use of the widely available ergonomic office products.

Poor posture is a habit. I treat many patients who have continual neck or upper back pain that is associated with slumping over a desk, working on the computer, and being on the telephone for hours. This does not even begin to account for the role of stress in causing back or neck pain. It is vital to remember that straining and re-straining your spine, day after day, has a cumulative effect. Repeated strain can cause your posture to become worse over time, which can lead to permanent damage. According to the March 3, 2000, *Mayo Clinic Health Letter,* "Neck Solutions," "Forward head posture (FHP) leads to long term muscle strain, disc herniations, arthritis, and pinched nerves." Other well-known effects of poor posture are spinal pain, headaches, mood problems, blood pressure problems, plus pulse and lung capacity problems.

Good posture improves our breathing, and good breathing improves the oxygen saturation in our blood. This increases alertness, and we will feel better all day. Poor posture is a habit that is formed over time. One of the easiest ways to get into the habit of good posture while sitting at a desk is to use the trick of the old Victorian grandmother: balance a book on your head! This will quickly show you how poor your posture actually is.

Fashion can also be detrimental to your spinal health. High-heeled shoes are popular with women, and it is doubtless they will always be popular. However, very high-heels that are worn every day force the lower spine into an awkward, unnatural position. High-heels slant the foot forward and bend the toes up, which causes the Achilles tendon to shorten, pushes the rump outward, compresses the lower back vertebrae, and causes muscle contractions. While high heels may make the female legs and derriere look great, high-heeled shoes strain the spine with every step. High-heels are biomechanically and orthopedically unsafe. Occasionally wearing high-heeled shoes may not be damaging to the spine; it is the cumulative strain of regularly wearing high heels that causes the difficulty. Heels can cause painful problems from the feet to the neck.

It is common to see adults carrying heavy purses or computer cases, and children toting heavy backpacks. People tend to carry too many items in totes, handbags, and briefcases, and they are unaware of the potential health risks associated with carrying excessive weight. Carrying a bag that weighs more than 10% of your body weight will affect balance and posture. This is especially serious when the bag is carried over one shoulder. Any one-sided activity, including sitting on a wallet, or shifting your weight to view a poorly placed computer monitor, trains the body to become asymmetrical. Any activity (such as carrying an infant on the hip) that causes a continual lean to the side, to counteract the weight, also causes the spine to curve in an unnatural manner. This causes the body to adapt its movement and to stress the musculoskeletal system, which subsequently develops into premature joint wear and makes the spine more susceptible to injury.

We spend almost one-third of our day sleeping. Mattresses that are too hard or too soft can create unnatural sleeping positions and overextend the spine or not properly support the spine. If you have spent the night in a hotel or at the in-laws on a very soft mattress, then you know that the next morning, you probably will wake up stiff and feeling like a pretzel.

A medium mattress has enough "give" to allow the spine to be in a naturally-aligned position when lying on one side, but it also has enough support, so as not to give too much, if you lie on your stomach. Sleeping positions can help with back pain. Test sleeping on your side with legs drawn toward your chest, and place a pillow between your knees. Test sleeping on your back with your knees supported and your legs elevated. These positions may also help for hip pain.

Sleeping positions are also a common cause of periodic neck pain and occasional headaches. Generally, it is better to use a pillow that does not force the head and neck position into an elevated angle. Feather pillows are preferred to extra-firm pillows, because they easily conform to the shape of the neck. However, there are also excellent memory foam pillows available.

Another area of concern includes lifting and twisting. Few of us have been taught how to lift objects. Even those who are required to lift heavy items at work often forget the rules for the safest way to lift once they are at home. Contrary to a common assumption, you can cause strain or injury to your back, or even cause a serious disc problem, if you twist your spine out of the correct position. This can happen if you are doing repetitive lifting. Smaller items, such as bags of groceries, babies, lap dogs, and flowerpots can cause spinal strains, stretching or tearing of the ligaments, and herniated discs. This is because the person is often twisting and lifting from an awkward position. Most people do not consider the implications of lifting while in an awkward position, or that there is a possibility that this could cause a severe problem. Even simple activities, done improperly, can cause spinal distortion and postural misalignment. Job duties that involve lifting, bending, or twisting repeatedly strain the back. This is a common cause of ligament strain in the back, and even a simple sprain/strain may take months to heal.

Lifting should not be attempted when the knees are locked, because this forces the spine to do all the work, and the spine is not designed to lift heavy objects. I advise patients to "keep the shoulders over the hips and over the heels." It is critical to keep the back straight and lift with the knees to avoid straining the back. Never lift heavy objects without help.

It is interesting that many of the men I see have just simply lifted something too large or too heavy for them. We have the perception that we are still 20 years old, and as we age, we rarely consider that our muscles and ligaments may not be in the same shape they once were. Even chores as common as gardening or movements as basic as getting up from the floor, can cause strain and injury in different areas of the body. Use common sense; if it looks too big and feels too heavy to lift without help, it probably is. Get some help!

## *Chronic Illness*

CHRONIC ILLNESSES AND long-term drug therapies inhibit the body's ability to heal. A limited healing capability can slow down and prevent recovery from back and neck pain, and lead to a long-term condition. Diabetes impairs healing. Steroids inhibit all aspects of the healing process. Chemotherapy and immune suppression drugs also impair healing, and there are many treatments and drugs too numerous to mention that can cause permanent change to the cells, systems, and organs.

A good example is my patient Jake. He owns a trucking company and has type 1 diabetes. At 59, he suffered from both neck and lower back pain. He had previously had a cervical spine fusion because he had degenerative disc disease causing pain in his neck and arms. After the fusion surgery, he was still experiencing the same pain. He refused to have low back surgery because he was now very skeptical. When Jake consulted with me, his chief complaint was pain in both legs. When he laid flat on his back, his legs would become numb and very stiff. He also had been diagnosed with diabetic neuropathy, which has symptoms of numbness and burning in the feet.

As someone affected by diabetes, Jake needed to monitor his glucose level, follow a specific diet, exercise regularly for his condition, and take medication or injections. Since diabetes inhibits the body's ability to heal, treatment time with the DRS Protocol™ sometimes needs to be extended. Jake was treated with the DRS Protocol™, and his back pain improved by 90%. I told Jake, prior to treatment, that the numbness and burning in his feet might not respond to treatment because it was probably related to his diabetic condition. However, Jake's numbness and burning completely went away because it was related to pressure on nerves instead of his diabetes.

A longer than normal recuperation period may be necessary for anyone with a chronic illness or medical condition. Treatments for cancer may affect the rest of the body and its capacity to heal, because chemotherapy and radiation therapies cause chemical imbalances as they work to eradicate or control a specific condition or inhibit cellular proliferation. In innumerable cases, the treatment will destroy metabolic enzymes and the immune function can be depleted. When functions are depressed and enzymes destroyed, these can have additional adverse effects on health and the body. This imbalance may influence how successful treatment of the spine will be and affect the time it takes to heal, since chemical imbalances slow down the body's response rates.

## Living with Pain

NO ONE WANTS to live with back or neck pain, but countless people do. The mere thought of having spinal surgery frightens patients, especially after they have experienced various ineffective or unsuccessful methods of treatment. Many more people in pain conclude, "If I just have surgery, all my pain and suffering will be gone. I believe this because this is what I have been told by my doctor." They believe that surgery is the sole answer. There is no partial commitment with surgery.

Some believe there are just two options: pain or surgery. Therefore, many back- and-neck pain sufferers will choose to continue dealing with pain medications and injections. Over time, these become less effective and must be increased. However, there may be a point when the doctor discontinues prescribing high doses of pain medication because he or she now feels the risks outweigh the benefits, and that includes the risk of abuse. The doctor must determine the patient's motive and intent. Because pain is subjective and pain cannot be seen, some of the determination is based on trust. Doctors have to be very aware of patients who exhibit addictive or "drug seeking" tendencies because of laws and abuse concerns. The bottom line may be that some patients will have to live with pain, and they are told, "Not everyone gets well."

Other recommendations for back or neck pain are anti-inflammatory medications, including nonsteroidal anti-inflammatories (NSAIDs) that commonly cause side effects such as ulcers and bleeding in the stomach or intestinal tract. Additional effects frequently experienced by patients on NSAIDs are nausea, vomiting, diarrhea, constipation, decreased appetite, rashes, dizziness, headaches, and drowsiness. These drugs may also cause fluid retention, leading to edema.

NSAIDs (except low dose aspirin) may further increase the risk of potentially fatal heart attacks and strokes. The risk may increase with duration of use and in patients who have the additional risk factors of heart and blood vessel disease. NSAIDs and Cox 2 inhibitors may cause secondary hypertension. Elderly patients are at greater risk for these side effects.

## *Types of Pain*

PAIN IS CONVEYED to the brain by a type of sensory nerve that only carries pain sensations, and these extend to every part of the body. No matter what kind of pain is present in the body, both sensory and motor nerves are involved. This combination of nerve response allows the pinpointing of the location of the problem, how serious the problem might be, and the nature of the problem (for example, whether it is a burn or a sharp pain). Pain can have a number of causes. Pain is more than just an absolute sign of physical injury; it is also a subjective interpretation.

There are several different levels or types of pain. One way to determine the level of pain a patient is experiencing is by using the visual analogue scale (VAS), which rates the severity of pain by starting at zero (0) for no pain, through ten (10) for unbearable pain.

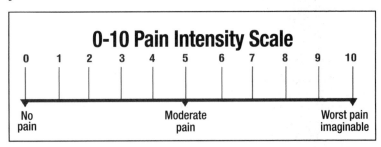

PAIN THAT IS immediately disruptive to a normal routine is referred to as acute pain. Acute pain usually is a result of actual tissue damage, such as a cut, bruise, or a broken bone. Other examples might include touching a hot object and burning your hand, catching your finger in a car door, or falling and scraping your knee on the pavement. Acute pain is a sudden and intense pain followed by a more aching pain. It is typically short and is resolved once the damage to the tissue is complete. However, if the pain persists over time, it can evolve into chronic pain.

Acute pain can also be associated with poor circulation or dehydration that might produce headaches or muscle cramps. Acute pain will normally diminish as the area is treated and the cause of the pain is removed or healed.

There is also a manifestation of pain known as referred pain patterns, which refers to pain that is conveyed by the internal organs and systems throughout the body to specific areas. A good example is pain felt in the left arm during a heart attack. Because signals from several areas of the body often travel through the same nerve pathways in the spinal cord and brain, pain from a heart attack can be felt in the neck, jaws, arms, or abdomen. A gallbladder attack may be felt in the back of the right shoulder.

Chronic pain is generally defined as pain that lasts beyond the normal time to heal from an injury. This is commonly thought of as four to six weeks, but some choose two to three months. Chronic pain, pain that persists once the body has healed, can be categorized into two large groups. The first group would include individuals who have a chronic disease such as osteoarthritis or degenerative disc disease and they will have ongoing pain because their disease and degeneration continually progresses. The second group includes those who have healed from the initial incident, but are not fully relieved of pain. The pain continues for no apparent reason. This can occur for numerous reasons, including the fact that the body may have compensated for the injury and that compensation now causes more pain. The body may have created scar tissue or adhesions, a natural mechanism for healing. However, the scar tissue itself may be pressing on nerves or within the scar tissue, there may be trapped nerve fibers and that is what is causing more pain. Chronic pain may also be the result of ongoing acute pain.

Long-term pain can also come from unknown causes, but this does not invalidate the patient's perception of pain. Pain occurs for a reason, and if it persists, there is a problem. One problem is that not all patients with similar conditions develop chronic pain, and it is not understood why some people develop chronic pain and others do not.

Pain from unknown causes that stimulates the nerves continually, if not resolved, can make the nerves more sensitive to pain. This becomes a downward spiral for those with back or neck pain. Over time, there is so much stimulation of the nerve in the form of pain, that it changes the nerve and causes ongoing pain, even after the problem has been resolved. It seems that the pain signal is sent to the nervous system, even without tissue damage. Also, there may not be a definitive point of pain. Perhaps the pain becomes the problem, as the nervous system is somehow misfiring and creating its own pain.

Neuropathic pain results from damage to, or dysfunction of, the peripheral or central nervous system, rather than stimulation of pain receptors. Diagnosis is suggested by pain that is out of proportion to tissue injury, and by dysesthesia (such as burning or tingling). In other words, rather than an injury causing pain, the nerves themselves are causing pain because they have become damaged and malfunction. The nerves become the source of the pain.

This category of pain, pain that persists when there is no apparent physical reason, has only been recently investigated seriously. This type of pain may indicate that the nerves carrying the pain signals to the brain may have been damaged from the previous injury. These damaged nerves continue to broadcast messages of pain to the brain even though the tissue damage has healed. The pain feels very different from pain caused by some sort of tissue damage. For most people, neuropathic pain feels like a severe shooting pain or a shooting, stabbing pain. It can radiate down the limbs and cause pain along the entire nerve path. This pain is often chronic and continues for months or years.

One of the unfortunate outcomes of chronic pain can be depression. It is now widely understood that pain does not just include a physical sensation. There is also a psychological element to pain, which is why it can be so complicated and difficult to treat. Pain affects the perception of the quality of life, which can lead to depression as the sufferer becomes frustrated and feels isolated by the inability to find relief.

Depression, fatigue, anxiety, anger, fear of additional injury, and stress or fear of losing a job are all chronic pain's emotional effects, and they interact in complex ways. Negative emotional feelings even affect the body's production of natural painkillers and increase the production of chemicals that amplify pain. The September 2004 issue of the *Harvard Mental Health Letter* states, "People with chronic pain have three times the average risk of developing psychiatric symptoms—usual mood or anxiety disorders—and depressed patients have three times the average risk of developing chronic pain." As the pain increases and becomes the focus, the individual who is suffering may experience symptoms of depression and anxiety.

The body and mind are closely linked, and when pain is involved, it can be much like a vicious circle. When we experience pain, the body responds to a perceived level of pain. I treat patients who exhibit a remarkably high tolerance for pain; I am amazed to see how much pain certain patients can tolerate while other patients are in agony from what would appear to be a less significant problem. This highlights why pain is so difficult to treat; there are no absolutes. Each individual perceives pain differently. There are no two patients, even if they appear to display the same exact findings on an MRI, X-ray, or other diagnostic tests, who will experience identical pain levels. Does this imply their pain is not real or is "all in their heads"? No, pain is a symptom of an underlying and sometimes serious condition, and it needs to be addressed. Unfortunately, many doctors may perceive certain patients' pain to be stress-related and treat the symptom as depression alone.

Pain not only affects the patient's life, it affects the lives of the patient's family members and friends as well. There have been cases where a patient has been in so much pain for so long that the family cannot remember what the patient acted like before the pain changed his or her personality. Sometimes, I tell a patient's spouse that I may even make the patient nicer, because as the pain subsides, they are able to focus on a healthier and more active life.

Many patients are surprised by how quickly their lives return to normal once the pain in their back or neck has been addressed. Even if someone has lived with pain for years or even decades, they can gain substantial improvement of mobility and be free from much, if not all, of the pain and discomfort. Mark is a good example of a person who had long-term back pain.

Mark came to see me when he was 47. He was a dispatcher for a trucking company. His chief complaints were low back pain and weakness in and along the outside of his left thigh. Mark's pain had started intermittently about ten years earlier, but for the last five years, he had been in continuous pain, which had sharply escalated in the last four months.

Mark's medical history was long and pockmarked with surgeries. Years before I saw him, Mark had a thoracic spine tumor removed when he was in his mid-twenties. This tumor was located on the vertebrae between the shoulder blades (T4-T7). Since the initial surgery, he had experienced weakness in his lower extremities and walked with a cane, as he had lost partial use of one leg. This altered his biomechanics and caused him to have both hips replaced when he was in his late thirties. Mark had been through years of pain and suffering of varying degrees.

Mark had already had the usual "conservative treatments" with injections and physical therapy for his low back pain and weakness, and he had been told by his orthopedist that he would need a lumbar spinal fusion. Mark was adamant about not having another surgery, but he needed help because he could not live with the level of pain he was experiencing.

After a thorough evaluation and examination, I concluded that the DRS Protocol™ would help Mark, with the understanding that the treatment period might be slightly extended due to his medical history. Mark's treatment proceeded cautiously so as not to aggravate any other medical problems. Mark had outstanding results: 100% resolution of pain. He was ecstatic. I treat him periodically to ensure he continues to maintain a pain-free life. *Surgery not Included.

To all patients with previous complicating histories, I emphasize the need for a realistic expectation of their outcomes. It is not reasonable for patients to expect to see improvement beyond what their condition was 20 years ago. However, the patients should expect to realize major improvement and pain relief. Each patient is different, and treatment must be customized to the individual's situation. Even two people who are experiencing similar problems may require different treatments, and they cannot expect to have identical outcomes.

It is important to seek treatment at the onset of pain. When a patient has suffered from pain for a long period, there is the potential for permanent nerve damage. Pain itself is not cumulative, however, the condition that creates the pain may cause cumulative or ongoing irritation to the nerve or the nervous system and that can cause permanent damage.

# CHAPTER 3

*The Patient Experience*

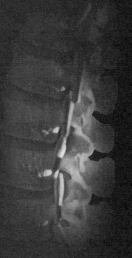

# CHAPTER THREE

*The Patient Experience*

W hen I was close to graduating from Parker College of Chiropractic, I attended numerous advanced educational courses, and during one, I heard a presentation given by Dr. John Ashton about a new technology, axial decompression, which could nonsurgically treat severe and chronic lumbar disc conditions. He was extremely impressed with the excellent outcomes produced through this new technology when used to treat chronic disc conditions, such as herniated disc or degenerative disc disease. At the time, Dr. Ashton told me that he believed axial decompression was going to become the future of treatment for chronic disc conditions. I felt he was right, and the thought of a treatment that would eliminate the need for surgery was exciting.

Axial decompression was developed by Allan E. Dyer, MD, PhD, who had served as Deputy Minister of Health in Ontario, Canada. The commercial name for the technology was VAX-D (vertebral axial decompression). Axial decompression, also known as spinal decompression, is a noninvasive treatment for chronic back pain conditions, and now neck pain from disc disease and facet joint disease.

My original training is in chiropractic care, and since my family publishes the leading national chiropractic magazine, *The American Chiropractor,* I have had many wonderful opportunities to meet and interview some of the foremost experts in their fields. One of those experts was Dr. Norman Shealy, a board-certified neurosurgeon who is a nationally recognized author and founder of the Shealy Institute in Springfield, Missouri, one of the most respected pain management facilities in the world. Dr. Shealy developed the TENS unit (TENS is an acronym for transcutaneous electrical nerve stimulation). A TENS unit is a portable, pocket-sized, battery-operated device that sends electrical impulses through the skin to block pain signals. Dr. Shealy also developed the DRS System for spinal decompression (DRS is an acronym for decompression reduction and stabilization).

Dr. Ashton was involved in consulting on the development of this new system. It was used to heighten the disc space of the vertebrae and relieve disc pain in the lumbar spine. The DRS System had some excellent new features that I favored over some of the limitations, at that time, of the forerunner, the VAX-D.

These spinal decompression tables relieved low back pain by decompressing discs, relieving direct nerve pressure, improving the absorption of nutrients into the disc, and rehydrating discs, thereby helping to improve disc structure.

Nonsurgical spinal decompression evolved from traction. Traction is a method of stretching the spine, in an attempt to reduce back pain. Traction has been used for years in physical therapy. Various methods have been used in producing traction from motors to weights, to inversion or tilt tables. One of the limitations with traction is how the force is applied. Traditional traction keeps the spine elongated for extended periods and uses constant force that activates a muscle-guarding reflex, which creates muscle spasm. However, spinal decompression provides controllable, distractive tensions to eliminate the muscle-guarding reflex.

Because a logarithmic wave of distractive force is applied in spinal decompression, the treatment allows the application of a greater amount of distractive force to the spine, both lumbar and cervical, than traction, without the side effect of the muscle-guarding reflex. The logarithmic application is important, as this allows spinal decompression to draw specific disc levels apart, which creates a negative pressure gradient from the inside to the outside of the disc, and allows the disc to be drawn back into its normal position.

When traction is applied, *only* the facet joints are drawn apart. Traction, over time, can increase the intradiscal pressure, rather than reduce the pressure. Potentially, this increased pressure can increase the patient's pain.

The significant lowering of the intradiscal pressure was confirmed in a study published in the *Journal of Neuroscience*, authored by Drs. Ramos and Martin. In this study, a cannula was inserted into the patient's lumbar disc space, and pressure transducers measured the pressure while the patient was treated on a VAX-D table.

A good visual of how a disc exerts pressure on the nerves is to think of a water balloon. If it is pressed on the top, the balloon expands equally on all sides beneath your hand. However, if it is then pressed on one side, the balloon bulges out to the other side. This is similar to how the disc behaves in the spine. Roll the balloon to the edge of a desk and it bulges downward. This is how a disc can put pressure on the nerves of the spine. Remove the pressure from the balloon and the balloon returns to normal. This represents the decompression of the disc.

The amount of pressure that the disc exerts on the nerves is quite small. A study from Colorado University in the mid-nineties showed 10mm mercury of pressure on a nerve (the weight of a dime) would reduce the effective functionality of a nerve by more than 60%. This is not a lot of pressure. I always tell my patients that I am not moving a refrigerator with spinal decompression just making minor changes to the spine, but it is enough movement to improve blood flow, alleviate pain, and help the body to heal. *Surgery not Included.

I started using the DRS System, a spinal decompression table, in the first years of my practice. I saw the ability to provide relief and improve the lives of thousands of patients who were suffering from severe back, and now neck pain, and did not want surgery. My practice was one of the earliest adopters of this treatment, and I quickly learned that the manufacturers build great equipment but rarely understand how to integrate that equipment into an active practice. I further realized that this was such a new treatment technology that manufacturers did not comprehend the full potential for spinal decompression for positive, long-term treatment outcomes for severe and chronic disc conditions.

After treating patients with spinal decompression for just a short time, I began developing my own treatment protocol, the DRS Protocol™, which is customized for each patient's individual needs. The DRS Protocol™ incorporates spinal decompression, chiropractic treatment, and other important elements including exercise and nutrition. The DRS Protocol™ manages the patient with specified treatment parameters, recorded benchmarking and tracking, reassessments and evaluations, and patient education. It is not limited to treatment on a spinal decompression table, but rather encompasses the complete patient experience. Treatment is specific to each patient's back or neck condition and is modified to fit the patient's individual needs.

My practice is located in Indiana, the heart of the Midwest. Historically, the Midwest is a very traditional and conservative area. This affects the patients' attitudes toward traditional medicine. Spinal decompression was a new treatment idea, and at first, there was some hesitancy in the medical community concerning the successful nonsurgical treatment of severe disc conditions.

Success was rapid with the DRS Protocol™, and the word about this successful nonsurgical treatment got around to other doctors. Some doctors began to call my office to inquire about the treatment and how to utilize it. Since then, I have provided advisory work for some manufacturers, and I have authored several articles on the subject.

Some surgeons went so far as to say I was crazy for expecting success in treating disc conditions with the conservative, alternative care I was offering, even when their own patients happily told them they had been successfully treated by me with DRS Protocol™.

Many patients readily understood the treatment concept, and spinal decompression easily made sense to them. Certain patients, such as engineers, farmers, and architects, completely understood the underlying concept, and while I treated them, they were trying to redesign some part of the equipment to enhance the appearance, structure, or even function.

After a few years, the proof was in the multitude of happy and satisfied patients who were able to live virtually pain-free without having to undergo any type of surgical or invasive treatment. It was not long before many medical doctors started referring their patients to my office first, rather than immediately to a surgeon. In some cases, the surgeons started sending patients to my office, and I was occasionally referred to as a friend. I was experiencing remarkable success rates with the DRS Protocol™. By this time, hundreds of patients had avoided surgery by being treated with the DRS Protocol™.

I had continued the discussion with Dr. Ashton about the future of spinal decompression. The potential for this treatment technology was tremendous. During the next few years, I had calls from doctors everywhere in the United States, asking for advice about treatment with spinal decompression. They had decompression tables in their offices, but could not determine how and when to use the treatment for maximum success. Dr. Ashton and I decided to work together to share the DRS Protocol™ with other doctors, so they could treat severe and chronic disc conditions, and to assure that they could achieve comparable results for their patients. Our consulting with medical doctors and chiropractors now helps patients all over the United States and certainly has reached more patients than I could ever treat in my personal practice. I have dedicated my life to helping as many patients as possible avoid surgery and live pain-free lives.

## *Surgical Outcomes: Side Effects*

THERE ARE UNFORTUNATE side effects for patients who have had surgery for disc conditions, especially fusion-type surgeries. These surgeries have a shelf life of two to five years, if even that, before the patient may begin to experience "failed surgery syndrome." This can occur because the bones or vertebrae are fused together, and the fused bones no longer move normally. This causes more movement and stress on the vertebral levels above and below the fused vertebrae, which leads to degeneration and more of the same problems in the areas adjacent to the fusion. A study published in the

July 2000 issue of *Spine* confirms that less than five years after spinal fusion, the adjacent vertebrae have disc narrowing or degeneration. Unfortunately, fusions are increasing (they doubled from 9% in 1993 to 19% by the year 2000), and while this rapid growth might suggest the surgery is effective, it has actually increased the need for repeated spinal surgery after spinal fusion. By 2000, the risk of repeat surgery in the first years after lumbar fusion was 40% higher than it was in 1993. Repeat lumbar spine operations are generally undesirable, implying persistent symptoms, progression of degenerative changes, or treatment complications (noted in "Increased Use of Spinal Fusion Hasn't Lowered Risk of Repeat Back Surgery," *Spine*, September 1, 2007).

For many years, studies have shown the poor long-term outcomes of spinal fusion, but many patients still believe that surgery will be a miracle cure. Unfortunately, surgery is not, which is why there has been so much research and so many clinical trials performed with replacement discs. It is well known that fusions are not a long-term cure and can cause many significant problems. In conversations with my patients, I have noticed that some surgeons are no longer rushing patients to surgery. What these surgeons are recommending is that patients wait until they can no longer bear the pain before even considering surgery.

After surgery for disc conditions of the back or neck, patients are often surprised and upset that they still have ongoing weakness and pain. This is frequently due to scar tissue, which is fibrous connective tissue created by the body for wound repair. If the scar tissue forms near a nerve root, which is a common occurrence in back or neck surgeries, this can cause pain. Nerve damage can be a direct result of scar tissue from the surgery. It happens to patients who have "successful" surgeries and yet continue to have pain. This can happen most often about 6 to 12 weeks after the surgery, and can follow an initial period of pain relief. The patient just slowly redevelops pain.

Even when a doctor says that scar tissue will be minimal, it can still be devastating, as it takes such a small amount of scar tissue to cause ongoing pain. Internal scar tissue can create adhesions and attach to internal structures causing pain. Scar tissue can be a debilitating side effect of surgery, because it can wrap around a nerve and more-or-less strangle or compress it over time. The pain caused by this can vary from mild to extreme, and it can cause constant or intermittent numbness and low back pain that radiates into the legs. This is known as sciatica, which can come on slowly, leading to an increase in intensity, and can even lead to a loss of coordination and restricted movement. In the neck area, a similar occurrence can take place. Some of the symptoms are pain down the arm, a weak hand grip, and numbness.

When scar tissue becomes a problem, surgical laser procedures are then recommended to remove the scar tissue, and this even happens after "successful" surgeries. Sometimes this needs to be redone every two to three years. Remember, it takes a minute amount (10mm) of pressure on a nerve to cause pain. The pressure would be similar to what you would feel if you balanced a dime on your fingertip. That is all the pressure required on the nerves in the spine to cause pain and reduce function. The problem of scar tissue contributes to "failed back surgery."

The issue of chronic pain associated with failed back surgery was reported as far back as 1994. The publication *Spine* featured an article entitled "Outcome of Lumbar Fusion in Washington State Workers' Compensation" (Franklin 1994), which stated: "Most patients reported that back pain (67.7%) was worse and overall quality of life (55.8%) was no better or worse than before surgery. Conclusions: outcome of lumbar fusion performed on injured workers was worse than reported in published case series."

Given these facts, the question is why surgery is recommended so readily and so frequently. The short answer is that surgeons perform surgery, that is what they do. A surgeon is a highly-trained doctor who has spent many years learning his or her craft and, by definition, specializes in the removal of organs, masses, and tumors, as well as other procedures using a scalpel. Surgeons also surgically treat disease, injury, and deformities. As a population, we could not live as long without them. They are trained in surgical intervention and have certainly performed many miraculous deeds.

A friend of mine, who is a surgeon, once told me that he had become tired of being ambushed by people at gatherings who wanted to discuss their medical problems, which usually ranged from minor to severe aches and pains, colds, and various other aliments. After growing very tired of being continually quizzed, he began to tell them the truth, and it stopped. When asked for his medical opinion, he would simply say, "I am a surgeon. That means that which I can't cut out, I do not know about." While it is a humorous story, it underscores the fact that surgeons are trained to treat surgically.

You may notice when you have an appointment with a medical doctor that he or she may do a very cursory examination, if any examination at all. In decades past, as much as 80% of a diagnosis was listening to the patient's history and examining the patient. Now, many doctors rely much more on tests, such as MRIs, CT scans, X-rays, and many others to develop a diagnosis. The reason is simple. Medical doctors, as part of insurance networks, are only paid for a 15-minute consultation and exam. Studies show that a doctor typically interrupts the patient's story after five or six minutes, and recommends medications. If this doesn't resolve the patient's problems, then on following visit the doctor will order diagnostic testing to verify the physician's first idea of what might be wrong.

Testing has come a long way, and insurance companies require objective tests before they will pay for treatment, rather than relying on the doctor's opinion. However, with respect to back pain, MRIs may not be conclusive or may show false positives and negatives. Pain cannot be measured with a test.

Some patients can have a disc condition that may not be definitive or appear to be minor on an MRI, yet it is not evident enough to diagnose. Either the report then reads "normal study," or there is no clinical correlation between the films and the patient's complaint. However, if a complete exam was performed and the findings reviewed, there would be clear indicators that the patient does indeed have a disc-related condition.

A disc condition may not be visible on the MRI, perhaps because the MRI was performed with the patient lying down, and there was no pressure on the disc causing the pain. At this point, the patient is often given some pain medications or anti-inflammatories, and told to come back if the problem gets worse. This scenario could be avoided if the proper examination was performed even when MRI results are inconclusive. Orthopedic and neurological testing can detect and allow treatment of disc-related problems early enough to avoid or limit the severity of pain later.

Treatment and healthcare decisions must be based on accurate diagnosis, but there can be errors in MRIs. Research published in the *Journal of Orthopaedic Surgery and Research* in October 2008 studied the accuracy of MRIs in detecting lumbar disc herniation. MRIs of 50 patients were evaluated. Of those, 28% who were positive for a disc herniation on the MRI did not have a disc herniation, and this was discovered during surgery. Another 33% of the patients who had a negative finding actually had a herniation ("The Accuracy of MRI in the Detection of Lumbar Disc Containment," October 2, 2008).

Have you ever wondered why many doctors do not discuss vitamins, herbs, and other natural remedies or complementary and alternative medical therapies (CAM), before prescribing medications, even though many medications have well-known and even potentially dangerous side effects? One explanation is the philosophical difference.

Allopathic doctors are traditional Western medical doctors whose general philosophy is to treat with drugs and surgery. Medical doctors, unless they specialize in CAM, have little or no training in nutrition and biological medicine. Medical textbooks have limited amounts of data on the benefits of nutrition and complementary therapies. These therapies may even be discouraged by their own medical boards as being nonconventional.

During their education, and every day they are in active practice, medical doctors are flooded with drug information. Drug representatives leave samples of the new "X" brand of antibiotic, pain medication, muscle relaxant, and antidepressant, while hoping to create a strong relationship with the doctor. This has to make the doctor wonder whether these drugs might be best for his or her patients. A doctor would be concerned about the safety, efficacy, and cost of a drug and its advantage over existing drugs. This requires reading the medical literature to compare the efficacy of the newer drugs to any of the older drugs on the market, which can be difficult because many studies for new drugs are only compared against a placebo and not an existing drug. This is an overwhelming amount of information for doctors to process, and because the pharmaceutical industry advertises directly to the consumer, this creates a demand for their product from individuals who have no idea if the drug is best for their situation. It is a big job for doctors to prescribe a drug, and the patient may influence some doctors' drug choices.

Ever wonder why health conditions are called a disease or syndrome, such as Alzheimer's disease, acid reflux disease, and degenerative disc disease? Any malady that is labeled a condition, syndrome, disease, or any other medical term cannot be treated in any way that is not approved by the FDA. This goes so far as to dictate that a medical professional cannot recommend a diet for someone affected by diabetes that has not been approved by the FDA. This FDA policy is the secret that gives pharmaceutical companies great power and influence in treatment and care.

Since almost every condition is now being named a "disease," this allows the pharmaceutical companies to develop a new magic bullet as a treatment for each problem, and prevents doctors from trying alternatives that might also work. The pharmaceutical companies are big businesses, and there is enough influence on doctors' preferences in prescribing to require legislation to stop improper influence on the medical professional who may not have the time or desire to investigate best medical practices for the patient.

The side effects of the influence of pharmaceutical companies on healthcare are a topic unto itself. However, patients need to become more inquisitive and take more responsibility for their own care. Every adult who can read and has access to a library or the Internet, should thoroughly research conditions, medications, possible treatment outcomes, and side effects, and not simply assume that the first recommended avenue of care is the only choice. Researching, at the very least, will lead to more educated questions. A patient who questions a medical diagnosis or treatment is not an aggressive patient, but a smart patient.

For those who have health insurance, their coverage and choices will be limited to the description and terms of their policies. Older indemnity policies allow more choice of providers and care. HMOs (health maintenance organizations) may cost less, but the patient's primary provider coordinates all care and imposes restrictions on the choice of doctors, facilities, and other ancillary care. The PPO (preferred provider organization) is an insurance organization in which member doctors and facilities work with a specific insurance company at negotiated, discounted payment rates. Of course, there is government insurance, Medicare and Medicaid, each with its own criteria, payment policies, and schedules. Doctors participating in insurance networks may find themselves in a quandary between what the best course of treatment for the patient is and what insurance will cover. In 2003, health savings accounts (HSAs) were legislated as an alternative to traditional insurance, allowing you to save money tax-free in an account for future healthcare needs. You control how the money in the plan is spent on healthcare expenses.

Doctors have a small amount of time to diagnose a condition or disease, and they are reimbursed according to insurance guidelines. The insurance industry has a massive computer database of the standardized times allowed per patient per condition. Insurance companies reimburse according to the patient's diagnosis and objective data. Regardless of whether the patient is hard-of-hearing, using a walker, or in need of a translator, the doctor will only be reimbursed for the standardized time. All doctors have to demonstrate is proof of a patient's problems in order to obtain insurance reimbursement. If a patient has a complaint, the doctor must offer a solution, and usually in the medical community, this is in the form of drugs or surgery. The easiest solution for the doctor is to do less extensive exams and rely on lab and diagnostic tests, and then refer patients to specialists.

All doctors wish to provide quality care (why else would we have studied and trained for so many years?), but the system is not always conducive to prescribing fewer drugs and carrying out the least invasive procedures. I am very pleased to be training chiropractors and medical doctors from all over the United States in the use of the

DRS Protocol™. This training offers doctors a treatment method for disc conditions that will provide a more complete understanding of the patient and his or her underlying condition. We can help patients with treatment and care without subjecting them to the potential side effects of drugs and surgery. And the results are replicable and amazing!

My principal desire for sharing my professional knowledge in *Surgery not Included is to inform as many people as possible, including doctors, patients, and patients' loved ones, about the DRS Protocol™, so that all doctors who offer spinal decompression can utilize it to the highest level and achieve the best results.

For well over a decade, and after having successfully treated thousands of patients, I am able to report that spinal decompression has been consistently effective. It works, and combined with the DRS Protocol™, the outcomes of treating spinal disc conditions are even more predictable and the success rates even higher. I have dedicated my professional life as a Doctor of Chiropractic to treating a category of patients who would have had surgery, according to conventional medicine. The DRS Protocol™ and spinal decompression have been proven successful, are steadily growing in public awareness, and are here to stay. There are no side effects—except that the patient avoids surgery, ongoing pain, and job loss.

As with any treatment, a patient's lifestyle and bad habits may affect results. With the DRS Protocol™, patients can continue a normal life and have significant relief depending on their history, age, and other underlying health conditions. *Surgery not Included.

Sharing this knowledge with both doctors and patients expands awareness of the option of an appropriate nonsurgical solution for low back and neck pain. The DRS Protocol™ can eliminate the need for surgery, but still allows surgery to be an option in the future, if necessary. However, when surgery is performed, the side effects from surgery, which can be reactions to anesthesia, unintended problems caused by the surgical "fix," or even naturally-occurring scar tissue—may *never* be undone.

My training is in chiropractic, which is the conservative management and treatment of health-related conditions and the human body. Spinal decompression melds with my healthcare philosophy and skill as a well-trained chiropractor: if interference is removed from the nervous system, the function of the nervous system will be corrected, which will therefore allow the body to heal itself naturally—given the appropriate conditions.

Prior to treatment with the DRS Protocol™ and spinal decompression, a patient may have considered other medical alternatives, including surgery. However, with the DRS Protocol™, we can provide predictable, successful outcomes for chronic disc-related conditions.

Not long ago, a friend's father was suffering badly from a chronic disc condition. I believed I could help the father through treatment with the DRS Protocol™. However, my friend's father had always taken conventional medical recommendations. He did not believe in alternative healthcare. Therefore, he just did not have the belief or the understanding of how the DRS Protocol™ could work for his condition.

This situation is very common and part of our human nature. We tend to gravitate toward that with which we are familiar, and we tend to take the word of people we consider to be experts, without question. What many people do not realize is that many common drugs came from nature. For example, before people started using aspirin, they chewed willow bark or boiled it and drank the tea to relieve pain. About 400 BC, Hippocrates, the father of medicine, advised chewing willow bark to ease the pain of childbirth. For centuries, people all over the world knew of its power to treat headaches, fevers, and inflammation. They were familiar with this remedy and knew Hippocrates to be a great physician.

My friend's father had a conventional, medical mindset about surgery when the idea of treatment with the DRS Protocol™ was suggested. He was only familiar with traditional care, and he was not familiar with this treatment. The father believed surgery was his only option because doctors had told him so. He just wanted to get it over with, and to be free from pain.

I saw my friend two weeks later and inquired about his father. His dad had not made it through surgery. He died on the operating table. This was a very tragic and sobering outcome. While the risk of dying during surgery is small, there is still a risk—and it could be completely unnecessary. Sadly, he is not the only person that I know of who has had a similar outcome.

Unfortunately, many patients are only offered certain treatment options, according to their insurance guidelines. One example is a sheriff that I previously treated with the DRS Protocol™. He had two herniated discs, and I treated him with great success.

Several years later, I asked a mutual acquaintance how he was doing. I learned that he had re-injured his back in the line of duty. Since his injury was work-related, Workers' Compensation directed him to seek care exclusively within the medical profession. Certain states have strong preferences as to the direction of care and enforce these preferences if claims are to be easily paid.

The sheriff went through the treatments within the back-and-neck pain pipeline, but he did not respond well to injections, pain medications, and physical therapy. Surgery was the next natural step and the preference of Workers' Compensation. Within a week of his surgery, he developed a blood clot (embolism) that moved to his heart and lungs, and he died. Again, it is fairly rare, but blood clots can be a surgical side effect.

In addition to the risk of blood clots, anyone who undergoes surgery is also at risk from the dangers of general anesthesia. There are many dangers of anesthesia, including symptoms as mild as a headache or as severe as an allergy or stroke. The brain can be affected by a lack of oxygen delivery during surgery, and bacteria such as the hard to control MRSA bacteria can be introduced into the body, causing infections that can be deadly.

## DRS Protocol™ Utilizing Spinal Decompression Is a Win-Win

THE MAJORITY OF patients that I treat have disc-related conditions. The noninvasive DRS Protocol™ utilizes spinal decompression to relieve pressure and allow the discs to receive the nourishment they need to heal. Treatment for patients with disc conditions will vary depending on their health plus the extent and severity of their problems. Even the most severe patients can be on their feet and back to work, within days. Surgery involves recovery time and medication, followed by physical therapy in some cases. In recent literature, it has been noted that physical therapy may benefit a post-surgical patient. However, it is not implemented enough. After surgery, there is significant downtime for patients, and it is often very difficult for patients to put their entire lives on hold.

The benefits of the DRS Protocol™, besides enabling patients to get better, are usually no downtime, no risk of anesthesia reaction, and no risk of death. An early study of the outcomes of patients undergoing spinal decompression reported that of 778 cases, 92% reported improvement (*Journal of Neurological Research*, Volume 20,

Number 3, April 1998). Since 1998, there have been additional technological improvements and patient management techniques.

It is important to understand that not addressing a disc problem can lead to other physical problems as well. When there is pressure on a nerve, feeling and strength will be affected, and function can be impaired. Pressure on a nerve can lead to visceral or organ-related problems, as well. Many women currently on medication for intermittent incontinence may have a minor disc-related problem. This problem is so prevalent that a friend, who is a chiropractor, discusses having a practice that is dedicated solely to incontinence.

Unfortunately, women may just tolerate back pain and incontinence. They may be resigned to the fact that the cause is age or weight, and simply assume that it is not curable. However, if the problem is disc-related, the DRS Protocol™ can improve their lives dramatically.

Another of the serious problems I treat is severe and debilitating headaches that limit patients' lives and keep them from being productive. Disc-related conditions in the neck may be the source of some headaches. Many patients may not realize that upper back or neck pain can be related to their headaches. The term "cervicogenic headache" means that the headache originates from the cervical spine or neck. Every part of the body is connected to the brain by nerves, and pressure on a nerve close to the spine frequently causes problems in another area. In many cases, when a patient complains of pain or numbness in the arms, the pain may originate from a disc condition in the cervical spine or neck. There are instances when a patient may have carpal tunnel symptoms in one or both hands (carpal tunnel is the compression of a key nerve in the wrist, causing numbness and pain), but it originates from a disc problem in cervical spine. Both this condition and headaches can be successfully treated with spinal decompression when they are disc-related.

Not being able to sleep is a frequent complaint of patients with disc conditions. They are constantly up and down all night, or awakened by pain and unable to get comfortable. Many have to sleep in a recliner, on the couch, or propped-up on pillows. Many patients who are in pain are forced to sleep in specific positions, such as in a sitting or reclining position. Some of my patients had not been able to sleep in the same bed with their spouses for years, yet they just put up with the pain because they did not want surgery. In addition, some medications can cause insomnia as a side effect. In addition to insomnia, patients may suffer from anxiety due to persistent pain, and one problem will aggravate the other. This may hinder coping and lead to feelings of guilt, which is yet another reason why some patients are unable to rest peacefully.

The nervous system controls every other system in the body. It is the master system. Irritation and inflammation of nerves can affect one or more areas of the body and even hinder the function of the digestive or circulatory system. In fact, this can affect any system of the body and cause pain in any extremity. There are so many variables affecting the symptoms patients may have that the list is literally endless.

## The Patient Experience

PATIENTS WHO COME to my office for the first time for treatment of back or neck pain may not know what to expect. To put my patients at ease, I explain to them that a complete medical history will be taken, a comprehensive examination will be performed, including orthopedic and neurological testing for clinical findings, and if they do not have current X-rays or MRIs available, then X-rays will be made.

Once I have completed the comprehensive evaluation, I sit down in conference with the patient and discuss my findings. When a patient is accepted for care, I discuss a definitive diagnosis, the term of treatment, and the expected outcome of the course of treatment. The majority of patients with back or neck problems, will see tremendous improvement with the DRS Protocol™.

Each patient has a specific and customized treatment plan, and treatment will vary with the severity of his or her problem. Each patient's treatment is based on his or her medical history and condition. Relief of symptoms may be achieved easily for most patients within the first few visits. However, some patients' conditions did not come about overnight. Whether their conditions are due to injury or degeneration, more treatment time may be required.

Patients who are seeking a magic bullet are going to be disappointed because their expectations are not realistic. Treatment is a process.

With the DRS Protocol™, the average course of treatment ranges from four to eight weeks, depending on the diagnosis and medical history. Even the patient who may require longer treatment time is usually eager to do so, when the cost of the DRS Protocol™ is compared to the cost of surgery—both financially and physically. There is the loss of time component when having surgery. Many times, a patient is not going to be able to work for weeks following surgery, excluding complications that could contribute to an even longer recovery. I am a firm believer in keeping people on their jobs whenever possible. The DRS Protocol™ is an excellent option with excellent outcomes.

Effective communication is a skill and is the key to patient confidence. Lack of clear communication can cause stress to the patient. A patient can be confused about the meaning of a diagnosis or treatment. My ability to communicate to a patient the meaning of the condition or diagnosis is a learned skill. My confidence in the DRS Protocol™ and discussing expected outcomes comes directly from successfully treating thousands of patients with chronic and severe disc conditions.

It is not unusual for a patient to start out being crabby. A few may be borderline belligerent at times. I understand pain can alter a person's personality, and I feel fortunate to be able to help a patient through the process. It takes someone who is trained and confident in patient care to see beyond someone's words and actions and understand the underlying causes. I treat patients who, because of their chronic pain, are difficult to deal with. Some feel their previous doctor discarded them; they had become high-strung due to pain. There is a small percentage of patients who cannot be helped by the DRS Protocol™. This may be due to other health issues or the fact that the patient's body may have a compromised ability to heal. If this becomes apparent, I discuss with the patient alternative conservative directions to pursue.

I stress that it is important to have treatment with an experienced doctor to achieve the highest success rates in spinal decompression with the DRS Protocol™. As you read the information presented here, I want you to know that there are successful alternatives to surgery. You do not have to live a life of pain. When you finish this book, I believe you will have the knowledge to find a treatment that provides long-term relief, with a doctor who can deliver the best results.

# CHAPTER 4

*The Desperate Patient*

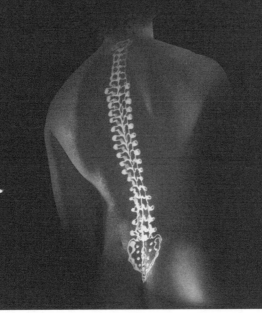

# CHAPTER FOUR

## *The Desperate Patient*

**P**ain is a powerful influence on life, and may cause people to do some interesting things. Patients struggling with chronic pain may have behavioral changes. Pain can cause people to say and do things out of the ordinary. Pain has the power to defy logic and override normal behavior. This may include taking large doses of over-the-counter pain relievers. Because OTC products are familiar, it does not occur to the patient that they can be dangerous drugs in large quantities.

Long-term use of NSAIDs (nonsteroidal anti-inflammatories) can stop the body from making prostaglandins, which are substances that help with some necessary physiologic functions, including protecting the stomach lining and regulating blood pressure. Long-term use of acetaminophen can cause liver or kidney damage due to its toxicity. Some patients may take OTC anti-inflammatories that contain the same active ingredients as other medications they take, which can cause an overdose even though the patient is taking the recommended dosage of each product. The FDA also reports that people who take NSAIDs and drink more than three alcoholic drinks per day may be at increased risk of gastrointestinal bleeding.

Some patients who are taking prescription pain medications report that they feel better when they take their pain medication and drink alcohol. This is a dangerous, and occasionally deadly, cocktail that any logical person would avoid. However, there are times that pain overcomes logic. Between 1999 and 2005, the number of overdose death certificates that mentioned poisoning by prescribed opioid painkillers went up by 83%.

Some patients really do not want a surgical procedure, but feel intimidated by or fearful of their doctor. In some situations, when a surgeon presses for a commitment to surgery, they can make a statement such as, "If we don't operate now, within a short time you will be in a wheelchair." I periodically hear reports of these types of comments from my patients. Another frequent comment reported is, "If we do not operate now, you will just continue to have the same problem, and in a year you will be worse." No matter how insistent a doctor is, surgery may not be the only option, unless there is an emergency.

It is just as depressing for a patient who is told by a surgeon not to do anything until the pain is unbearable. Other patients live in a state of constant denial, ignoring the pain and refusing to do anything about it until they can no longer live with the pain. They are usually unaware that a nonsurgical treatment is available, and would rather ignore their pain than face the prospect of surgery.

Antidepressants are frequently prescribed for patients suffering with back pain. This is because living with constant pain can create depression. Once a patient admits or demonstrates depression, the doctor may believe that the depression is contributing to the pain. In the past, antidepressants were more frequently prescribed as a short-term treatment of back pain. One theory behind using antidepressants for the treatment of low back or neck pain is that low doses of tricyclic or tetracyclic antidepressant medicine may increase the level of certain chemicals in the brain, which can upset the chemical pathways for pain. Several studies show that while antidepressants may be beneficial for pain in the short term, it is unclear how they work. They may also help patients sleep. The dark side of these medications, as with many pharmaceutical products, is that they have side effects that can be as mild as dry mouth or as serious as suicidal tendencies.

Pain often rules the lives of patients with disc conditions. Severe back or neck pain may limit the ability to do something as ordinary as picking up a glass of water, let alone working without pain. I treated a patient who reported that a surgeon who had evaluated him recommended a change in profession. A simple question: how easy is it for anyone to change a profession or career? Unfortunately, many people suffering from pain are forced to leave successful careers because they cannot perform the required duties.

If a patient cannot go shopping or enjoy outings to church or other activities, the result is a limited lifestyle. Social isolation and frustration may also result, as physical activity is limited. It is difficult to know all the thoughts, fears, and perceptions at work in patients' heads. However, I do know that dealing with constant pain is fatiguing and mentally draining. Pain medications can cause drowsiness and result in severe fatigue along with the inability to perform normal activities.

At the beginning of care, I make a point of talking with patients' spouses. I often mention that I am going to make their spouse "nice" when we are all done with treatment. Many times, a spouse will look at me and say something to the effect of, "Well, if you can do that,

Dr. Busch, any treatment would be worth it!" Invariably, while the patient is going through care, I have the opportunity to bring up the subject again and ask if the spouse is now nicer. The common response is that the spouse is nicer, and with less pain is able to get around to do things she or he has not been able to do in years. A problem with people suffering is they frequently make the people who care for them pay for their discomfort.

Individuals in pain can be angry, withdrawn, and downright mean. Pain can lead to resentment on the part of family and friends as well. It is very difficult to watch a loved one in pain and as the patient's personality becomes more extreme, it can be difficult to understand.

Pain has the power to prevent people from socializing and establishing new relationships, and pain can damage existing relationships. Not only does pain create moodiness and emotional swings, it can also limit activities and leave a spouse either to do things alone or suffer the same limited life. Pain can prevent a grandparent from picking up a grandchild. Older people feel stripped of dignity and lose the expectation of achieving a higher quality of life. Pain can control every aspect of a person's life.

## *Removing the Pain*

AS A CHIROPRACTOR, I deal with people who have varying degrees of disc conditions and levels of pain every day. Herniated discs, degenerative disc disease, and even stenosis, cause pressure on the nerves and inflammation, and these are the cause of much of my patients' pain. In some cases, these conditions will respond to chiropractic care. These problems are different from a subluxation, which is the imposition of bone putting pressure on a nerve and affecting the way that nerve functions. However, a condition resulting from pressure on the nerves from severely herniated or degenerative discs can be more difficult to treat. I treat these conditions with the DRS Protocol™.

Pressure on a nerve can affect the way any organ in the body works, and this is demonstrated effectively with sexual dysfunction. Sometimes, the pressure on the nerves in the low back (L3-4) may make it very difficult, if not impossible, for a male to achieve an erection or for a female to achieve an orgasm. This is because as the nerves exit the spine they are connected to an end organ. This end organ is innervated (connected to the nervous system by nerves) as are the muscles in the same area. If everything is communicating properly, organs function correctly. If there is a lack of communication between the brain and the body or organ due to pressure on the nerve, this can certainly affect the way those organs function, as well as muscle strength and the sensation of the skin.

About five years ago, a patient came to me for evaluation. He had complaints about his back and some leg pain, and he brought in an old MRI. After his examination and X-ray, I informed him that he had a herniated disc, and I discussed the possible outcome of treatment with the DRS Protocol™. Soon after beginning care, during a re-evaluation, the patient mentioned that his wife was very happy with his progress. Of course, I asked him why, and he said that prior to beginning care, and for the last several years, he had difficulty performing in the bedroom.

During his initial exam, he had never mentioned this as a problem, and he had never addressed his erectile dysfunction (ED) because he was embarrassed. He told me that after treating him for one week, he noticed that the problem was resolved, and he was able to "perform" whenever desired. He and his wife were both elated with the results!

As intimacy decreases, relationships suffer. Many patients suffering with chronic pain perceive this as a lack or loss of personal control. Something that may also happen, because of a patient being in pain and feeling out of control, is the desire to take more control over other aspects of life. I frequently notice patients trying to control their children or spouses as a result of their pain. It is a very complex situation, and every doctor should be aware of this possibility.

There are some situations in which patients may feel pain is helpful in their relationships. I recall a humorous story of a patient, Sandy, who was instructed to eliminate any activities that might aggravate or increase her low back pain. For two weeks, she was to discontinue activities such as raking, vacuuming, and bending to empty the dishwasher. A DRS assistant working with Sandy noted that she was reporting 100% improvement with normal activities. However, Sandy cautioned the assistant, "Shh, I haven't told my husband that I can do any work like that." As far as her husband was concerned, it took quite some time for Sandy to return to normal activities.

The story about my next patient is quite the opposite. I have a memorable 86-years-young patient named Miss Betty who experienced a major flare-up as a result of a fall. She had a herniated disc that affected her so badly she was forced to use a wheelchair. I did not know it until later, but because of her dependence upon a wheelchair, she did not want to be seen in public using a cane, walker, or wheelchair. Betty gave me a hard time about getting her well again because she was not going to church until she was out of "that chair" and was not going to use the walker.

Her family wanted Betty to get a second opinion, so an orthopedic surgeon saw her when she was halfway through her care at my office. (Sometimes, improvement takes a little time if there's a chronic degenerative condition complicated by a herniated disc.) The second opinion from the surgeon was that Betty needed surgery. Betty said no, even though the doctor told her she would never be able to walk without a cane and she certainly was not going to be able drive again. I treated Betty just the other day for supportive care, and yes, she drove herself to my office, and she was walking without a cane. *Surgery not Included.

Embarrassing problems that are usually associated with age, such as wheelchairs, canes, walkers, aches and pains, and problems with incontinence and impotence, can contribute to patients feeling much older than they actually are. All of these problems can lead pain sufferers to believe that their life has been destroyed, and they cease to dream of getting better. They stop growing and developing, and merely exist. For some patients, their pain becomes their identity. We have all known people like this. Their whole life is framed in pain. Chronic pain is not a passive episode, instead pain becomes life. It can be difficult for people in pain to relate to others when all the others hear is the account of their pain, their doctor visits, and how awful their life is. They may even have a feeling of grief about losing their former identity and life due to the pain. Moreover, while some may be relatively young, their lives have been fast-forwarded by decades. They may even be living as if death is imminent—when it is not, and it does not need to be this way.

## *Dealing with Doctors*

PART OF THE frustration for patients is the experience of going through the back-and-neck pain pipeline. Even though I know many kind and capable doctors, the patients' frustration is that they have not only been told their only option is surgery, but they have already gone through the pipeline before and they know what the next step is. Everyone knows someone who has had surgery with less than a successful outcome. Invasive procedures carry their own side effects. I believe that if most people were knowledgeable about their treatment options, they would rather choose conservative care, such as the DRS Protocol™.

Many patients are familiar with the idea behind chiropractic care and want a holistic treatment approach that provides the body with an environment to heal itself. However, I have seen many patients who have not responded to previous chiropractic care, and were told that surgery was their only option. Since they do not want surgery and they are not confident that chiropractic will help, they just get right back into the back-and-neck pain pipeline to try it again with pain medications, physical therapy, injections, and perhaps more extensive and painful diagnostic testing. Alternatively, they do not do anything, and in many of those cases, they may feel misled and at a standstill.

Even after another round of unsuccessful treatment, patients are often told they still have a choice: they can have surgery, just as the surgeon had originally recommended, or they can choose not to have surgery—but they'll be back in this same place with these same choices, no matter what. At that point, they may be released to fend for themselves, or may be sent for pain management and given continued pain medications. If necessary, they may have implantations of a spinal cord stimulator or a pain pump.

When patients decide against surgery, they can feel hurt and resentful if they have a sense that they are being talked down to by the physician. Patients are not ignorant for wanting conservative care, and I believe that often the medical doctor does not understand the validity or efficacy of a conservative treatment such as the DRS Protocol™ (although I am training more and more medical doctors around the nation). Because they do not understand the alternatives, they do not recommend them, and many still are not aware of spinal decompression and the DRS Protocol™. Sometimes, surgeons intimate that the patient is not making an intelligent decision. That may end the decision-making cycle, and the patient will break down and follow the surgeon's recommendation, even if they do not like the decision.

If the patient refuses surgery, or if the back or neck surgery fails, the next referral may be to a pain specialist, a doctor who has acquired the necessary didactic and clinical skills to evaluate and treat pain appropriately and effectively. This doctor will usually continue to prescribe pain medication, step up the dosage, or prescribe stronger medication to control the pain. Some pain specialists prescribe the latest drug—not necessarily the best drug or one that has not even been studied for the patient's type of pain.

Some doctors may prescribe medications that are "off label," meaning they are used for a purpose for which the drug has not been studied or tested. In some cases, this may help the patient feel better, but it is also possible that the patient will have an entirely different set of side effects and pains as a result. Unfortunately, many of these drugs are addictive and very powerful. They can alter the patient's personality and at times alter mental or physical function.

There are limits to how much pain medication is safe to take, and a pain specialist must monitor dosages. Accidental overdoses happen on a regular basis. Over a 20-year span, fatal medication errors (FMEs) were listed as the cause of death on more than 224,000 death certificates (*USA Today,* July 2008). That is a tremendous number of deaths each year due to accidental overdoses or fatal drug interactions.

During surgery, the nerves can be irritated, bumped, and stretched, which can cause many unintended consequences such as long-term back pain, loss of movement or sensation in the legs or feet, loss of bowel and bladder function, and permanent spinal cord injury (although rare).

Following surgery, patients are often angry with their doctor, even if they have a great doctor, because they may be worse due to scar tissue and possible nerve damage.

Yet, there are times when surgery is necessary, regardless of the inherent side effects. For instance, surgery is required immediately when a patient is diagnosed with Cauda Equina Syndrome (a condition where there is loss of bowel control or bladder function accompanied by severe lower back and leg pain). However, those circumstances are rare. While the prevalence of surgery for moderate-to-severe disc-related conditions is very common, patients may have a much better outcome with noninvasive treatments such as the DRS Protocol™.

Almost everyone knows someone who has had failed back-or-neck surgery, or whose outcome was not as successful as expected. One reason is the involvement of the nervous system. Spinal surgery is not the same as having a knee or hip replaced. With knee replacement, the normal expectation is to live a relatively pain-free life. Spinal nerves are highly integrated into the structure of the spine, and surgically altering the structure that protects and supports those nerves and the spinal cord can have a long-term and detrimental effect on the patient.

This is one of the critical reasons I feel it is absolutely necessary to perform a comprehensive physical exam and thorough case history, along with orthopedic and neurological exams. For those rare instances when surgery is necessary, it is imperative that I find this out immediately and that the patient knows as well. If it is the rare case I cannot treat, I immediately refer the patient to a specialist.

Conversely, for the many people with disc conditions that I can help, I want them to know that they do not have to face invasive intervention to find help and relief. They should know as soon as possible that they do have a successful alternative—"Surgery not Included.

## *Patients with Health Issues*

MANY PATIENTS ASSUME that treatment with the DRS Protocol™ is only appropriate if they are in otherwise excellent health. Fortunately, this is not true, and I have a great deal of success with patients who have a range of health issues. The following are some of the more common conditions that I see in my practice.

## *Osteoarthritis*

OSTEOARTHRITIS, ALSO KNOWN as DJD (degenerative joint disease), is a type of arthritis in which there is a breakdown and eventual loss of the cartilage between the joints. It does not happen overnight; it is a slow process of the cartilage breaking down. When arthritis occurs in the spine, it is called DDD (degenerative disc disease). The discs between the vertebrae degenerate and decrease the height of the discs. This can cause irritation and pressure on a nerve, resulting in pain, and can cause irritation to the facet joints on the backside of the spine as well. The following are common symptoms: aching joints after physical activity, stiffness and loss of flexibility after getting out of bed or sitting for long periods, and a crunching feeling or sound or a grinding sensation when a person turns the head or moves any other joint.

This type of arthritis is the most common, affecting more than 20 million people in the United States. Osteoarthritis becomes more common with age. By age 65, 50% of the population has evidence of osteoarthritis, and it tends to affect more women than men. A genetic component contributes to some cases. Other factors are obesity, poor nutrition, lack of exercise, changes in posture, and disease.

I see many patients with this condition, and as the baby boomers age and obesity increases, I expect to see many more. Osteoarthritis can also be the result of an old injury that caused damage to a joint or the joint capsule. Over time, this can create a change in the movement of the joint and damage the bone around the joint. Osteoarthritis can also result from improper movement of a joint over many years. The improper movement continues to put an abnormal stress on that joint, and that leads to degeneration.

## *Osteoporosis*

OSTEOPOROSIS IS A condition of decreased bone mass, which leads to risk of fracture due to the fragility of the bones. Anyone can develop this disorder, but it is more common in older women. As many as half of all women over 50, and a quarter of all men in that same age bracket, will break a bone due to osteoporosis. The latest information regarding osteoporosis is that there is no single cause, but some causes are heredity, ethnicity, lifestyle, side effects of disease, and medication. Certain medications, including steroids such as Prednisone, a corticosteroid, inhibit absorption of calcium in the intestine. Immunosuppressant drugs may also cause bone loss.

Due to the inherent problems associated with this disorder, a doctor must be aware of the patient's bone density. Bone density is checked through a Dexa scan that gives a risk score. As the disease progresses, a person's bones are very fragile and very susceptible to compression fractures in the thoracic and lumbar spine as well as the hips. In advanced stages, simple bending can cause a compression fracture.

The DRS Protocol™ is very gentle, and an osteoporotic patient can achieve good results and substantial pain reduction. This type of patient is closely monitored and has frequent re-evaluations.

# *Diabetes*

VERY SIMPLY, DIABETES is a disease characterized by high blood sugar. There are two major types of the disease. Type 1 diabetes is usually diagnosed in children and young adults and was previously known as juvenile diabetes. Type 1 diabetes is an autoimmune condition. The body does not produce insulin, which is a hormone that is required to convert sugar (glucose), starches, and other food into energy. The result is high blood sugar, which at abnormally high levels over time can damage tissue and organs and even cause death if left untreated.

Type 2 diabetes is the most common form. With Type 2, either the body does not produce sufficient insulin or the cells do not recognize the insulin. Type 2 causes glucose to build up in the blood instead of going into cells. This can cause two problems: cells will be starved for energy, and over time, high blood glucose levels may hurt the eyes, kidneys, nerves, or heart.

It is essential to know the extent of a patient's diabetes and to know how well it has been controlled before treatment. Many patients are able to manage diabetes by simply following a diet and by exercising. Other patients affected by diabetes may require daily medication, along with dietary and exercise recommendations, and others may require insulin.

Diabetes suppresses the immune system, slows healing, and can directly affect the nerves. Patients with diabetes may feel numbness, burning, and pain in their extremities due to a condition called diabetic neuropathy. Diabetic neuropathy is a common complication and the symptoms can have a range of manifestations, including almost no symptoms at all. However, the symptoms can also be quite severe and include tingling and numbness in the extremities, weakness and wasting of the muscles in the hands and feet, problems with urination, and gastrointestinal problems.

Neuropathy is nerve damage resulting from high blood glucose levels and low oxygen levels. Another factor is the length of time these levels have been affecting the nerves. Overtime, the damage will increase.

Problems can occur in every system, including the digestive tract, heart, and sex organs. When treating patients who have diabetic neuropathy, it is important to differentiate between the disease process and a disc-related condition. This can be very difficult. When a diabetic patient presents with a neuropathic condition, the exam findings may include diminished sensitivity plus complaints of numbness and tingling or burning.

Diabetic neuropathy will not respond to treatment with the DRS Protocol™. Because people affected by diabetes have a suppressed immune system, this also means that the patient may not respond as quickly to treatment. Therefore, I discuss these limitations with patients affected by diabetes. Having said that, most will have great results from the DRS Protocol™. With surgery, there is some evidence that they will have more complications than other patients following lumbar fusion. The next story is a particularly memorable one of a discouraged patient with diabetes.

John was a 58-year-old with diabetes, and he was on a downward spiral. He had not monitored his diabetes closely, and he certainly did not watch his diet. While his diabetes was under control to a degree, he was not in good condition. John was 75 pounds overweight, and he had been in pain with a lumbar disc condition for 10 years. He was suffering with low back pain along with pain in his legs and feet. Diabetic neuropathy contributed to his foot pain. He was cantankerous and appeared to have given up hope.

As I talked with John about his diabetes and treatment for his disc condition, I impressed upon him the point that treatment would progress much faster and he would have the best results if he took better care of himself. With an eye roll and a shrug, (it is difficult to exercise when you have back, leg, and foot pain), John agreed to try to take better care of himself, and then he started treatment with the DRS Protocol™.

Within two weeks, John was feeling noticeably better. His low back pain was diminished, and his leg and foot pain were almost resolved! It was not diabetic neuropathy after all. This gave John a lot of hope. He told me that because his foot pain was almost gone, he was excited, and he really did feel like taking better care of himself. Before treatment with the DRS Protocol™, he did not see any benefit in watching his weight or his diet, since he was in pain all the time anyway. It took some improvement and a reasonable effort on his part, to convince him to continue with healthier habits. Then his improvement accelerated.

Patients living with chronic conditions may not feel that there is hope for improvement. However, relieving the pain from their disc conditions can be a reality and can change their lives.

## Heart-Related Conditions

HEART CONDITIONS INCLUDE coronary heart disease, arrhythmia, heart valve disease, cardiomyopathy, and aorta problems. Many heart conditions can lead to heart attack and stroke. I have treated many individuals who have had some type of heart-related condition.

Patients who have had heart attacks usually have no issues at all in undertaking treatment with the DRS Protocol™, though a heart attack can cause extensive damage to the heart muscle and leave the patient with general weakness. The DRS Protocol™ can help with reducing pain and alleviating weakness due to pressure on the nerves of the spine. Of course, any general weakness brought on by damage from the heart attack will not be improved.

Many heart attack patients who have blockages in the arteries will have stents surgically placed to improve blood flow to the heart. A stent is a wire mesh tube that is implanted in an artery using an angioplasty procedure. Stents are inserted through an artery, and this incision must be allowed to heal at least five days prior to treating with spinal decompression. These patients will achieve very good results with the DRS Protocol™.

In the United States, strokes are the number one cause of disability and the third most common cause of death in adults. Strokes are associated with excessive weight, high blood pressure, heart disease, diabetes, and a family history of stroke. Other factors are unhealthy lifestyles and habits such as smoking, poor diet, and lack of exercise. Strokes are caused by a blockage or lack of blood supply to specific areas of the brain, which can leave lasting neurological problems. These problems may include weakness, difficulty moving, and even paralysis.

A patient who has had a stroke must be evaluated and examined carefully to be certain the problem is disc or spinal nerve related. The DRS Protocol™ cannot improve any permanent damage caused by a stroke, but disc-related pain can be helped, and that will improve the patient's mobility. Stroke patients often experience a change in gait or function due to weakness in limbs on one side of the body. These changes can cause the spine to twist into unnatural positions as the patient tries to compensate for the biomechanical deficiencies that cause pain. This pain, if determined to be from a disc problem, can be treated by the DRS Protocol™, and will help improve function. The expectation for improvement is similar to that of any other patient.

## *Transplant Patients*

ONCE VERY RARE, there are now thousands of people who have had organ transplants. Most transplant recipients must stay on anti-rejection drugs for the remainder of their lives to ensure their bodies do not reject the transplanted organ. These drugs suppress their immune system. A patient with a transplant is treated as any other immune-suppressed patient. They are evaluated and monitored carefully.

When it is determined that the condition is appropriate for treatment with the DRS Protocol™, treatment is begun and the patient's progress is followed closely. In my practice, I have treated two heart transplant recipients and several kidney transplant recipients, all with excellent results. With a transplant patient, it is very important to be aware of all medications that the patient is taking. I do not introduce any nutritional supplements without the advice of the transplant specialist. While transplant patients may require increased treatment time, it has been my experience that they respond very well.

## *Amputees*

I HAVE TREATED many amputees. Lower extremity amputations often affect the spine because the amputation naturally affects how the amputee bears weight. The gait and biomechanical function of an amputee is changed forever. Change of structure and function puts additional pressure on the spine and over time will cause degeneration of the spine and surrounding structures that are overstressed.

A patient of mine, Dave, has a dramatic story with a great outcome. Dave was involved in a terrible motorcycle accident. He eventually lost his leg just above the knee, and he was fitted with a prosthetic leg. As he was recovering and going through physical therapy to learn to use his new leg, he experienced significant pain. He was told that this was normal and that he was experiencing phantom pain. Phantom pain is a common occurrence in which the nerves send signals to the brain so that the brain perceives the amputated limb is attached, and the patient continues to feel pain. Nothing Dave tried successfully alleviated the pain.

Dave came for evaluation on the chance that I could alleviate any pain. His examination was difficult to perform. The normal orthopedic maneuvers used for evaluation had to be altered due to his missing leg. Within the first week of treatment with the DRS Protocol™, he was amazed at how well his body had responded. He stated that 80% of the time, he did not feel any pain in his low back or leg, and by the end of the course of treatment, his pain was completely gone. He was not actually experiencing phantom pain. Dave's real problems were related to his new prosthetic leg. The problem was two-fold: first, he was walking on an unsteady and uneven foundation. The prosthetic leg was not even with his other leg, and therefore he was functioning with legs of different lengths. His orthopedic doctor corrected this part of the problem. The second problem was that as he learned to walk with his prosthetic leg, his natural gait was altered, and this biomechanical change added to the problem.

Dave's story highlights the fact that there may be more than one answer when dealing with the human body. He no doubt originally had some phantom pain, as many amputees do, but a large source of his pain was the result of a degenerative disc condition. Prior to his accident, Dave had a degenerative disc that I had successfully treated, and since his accident, he had new symptoms. His major symptoms were resolved by treating Dave with the DRS Protocol™. Dave is still doing well. *Surgery not Included.

## *Mental Degenerative Diseases*

I FREQUENTLY TREAT patients who are suffering from different degrees of Alzheimer's or dementia. It is estimated that five million people in the United States are currently afflicted with Alzheimer's, which is considered the most common type of dementia.

Alzheimer's destroys a person's brain cells, and it is slowly incapacitating. Over time, it is fatal and is currently the sixth leading cause of death in America. Dementia is a general term used to describe cognitive degeneration stemming from a variety of reasons. Many people with dementia have Alzheimer's, but not all. Vascular dementia is caused by a narrowing of the blood vessels, thereby causing the blood supply to be cut off from the brain. The effect is similar to that of a stroke.

Both Alzheimer's and dementia are progressive neurological diseases of the brain that lead to impairment in memory, judgment, decision-making, speech, and orientation to surroundings. People with these diseases can exhibit strange behavior, and they can easily injure themselves or cause damage to their back and neck. Even those who are largely mentally incapacitated will still respond to treatment, and they certainly deserve to live free of pain.

Of course, with patients who suffer with Alzheimer's or any form of dementia, I require that a family member who is in charge of healthcare decisions be present for any treatment decisions.

Parkinson's is another degenerative disease seen in patients generally over 50 years old. The disease may start with mild tremors in one hand, then as the dopamine-producing cells in the brain degenerate, uncontrollable tremors occur in various parts of the body. Patients will have a change in gait, and their arms do not swing while walking, which causes them to lean forward and may even cause them to fall.

Part of the progression of Parkinson's is diminished reflexes. Therefore, if the patient is continually leaning forward or stooping over, this creates back and neck pain because the body has altered biomechanics. Patients with Parkinson's will also respond well to treatment for disc-related conditions.

Many symptoms of degenerative neurological diseases such as Parkinson's, Alzheimer's, dementia, and others will not directly respond to the DRS Protocol™. The DRS Protocol™ will only alleviate pain in the back and neck related to disc conditions, and it will not slow the progression of the disease.

Patients with other preexisting health conditions will benefit from treatment with the DRS Protocol™ for the appropriate neck and back conditions. It only takes a short time to do an evaluation that can determine if a patient is a candidate. My mind always returns to my friend who assumed his father was not in good enough health to have treatment and his father did not believe in alternatives. His father opted for surgery instead and died during that surgery. I cannot help but believe that had he decided on a nonsurgical treatment, he would have had many more good years with his family. Never assume someone is not a candidate for the DRS Protocol™ until a qualified evaluation has been performed.

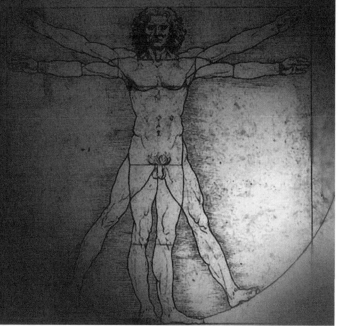

# CHAPTER 5

## Other Treatments

# CHAPTER FIVE

## *Other Treatments*

**M**any patients, prior to coming to my office, have already undergone other types of treatment for back or neck pain. Often, treatment is considered effective even though only short-term relief is the expected outcome. Other treatments are not effective at all.

Long-term relief is statistically not the rule when dealing with conventional treatment of herniated discs. I want to discuss some of the treatment options as they may be some you have tried or heard about, and either had a good experience or a disappointing one. I would like to encourage you that no matter what your previous experience with any other treatment was, you can still have a good experience with spinal decompression when DRS Protocol™ is used.

Much nonemergency medical information is obtained from people we know other than the doctor: the neighbor, the friend at church, or the person at work. That is the method we use to find the best sales, the favorite restaurants, and the movies that are worth seeing. People often share medical advice. This may lead to misinformation about medical conditions and which treatment is right for you. This word-of-mouth is also how we can find doctors that are liked. However, it does not excuse us from becoming knowledgeable enough to ask competent questions and find the right care. Just because your Aunt Tilly suffered back pain for years, does not mean that you have to suffer!

## Late-Night Remedies

WHO HAS NOT occasionally sat up late at night watching infomercials and been tempted to order the Ginsu knives just in case they are as great as they advertise? Back or neck pain sufferers often have insomnia, and they frequently find themselves channel surfing on late-night television. When patients are dissatisfied with medical options or their own personal treatment outcomes, or perhaps they have a deep-seated fear of doctors, they may start buying products and programs that seem to offer hope to solve their chronic problem. In addition, many patients feel lonely and abandoned because of their problem, and to them, watching an infomercial is like joining a family. These offers may include vitamin programs, exercise regimens, massage chairs, gravity boots, and various inversion tables or mechanical devices that purport to relieve back pain. Sometimes, patients do experience temporary relief in certain circumstances, but it rarely lasts long, and there is a very real potential to aggravate the problem rather than cure it.

The majority of the time, these products do not do a thing to improve the situation, and the patient is still in pain, albeit a little lighter in the wallet. It is important to note, there is a reason infomercials state that *individual results may vary:* they vary widely!

# *Drugs*

PATIENTS WILL OFTEN try to alleviate a pain problem themselves by taking larger doses of over-the-counter medications. This includes NSAIDs (nonsteroidal anti-inflammatory drugs) such as aspirin, ibuprofen, or ketoprofen.

Once a patient decides to see a doctor, the first step in alleviating back pain for most medical professionals is to prescribe pain medications and/or anti-inflammatories. These may include steroids. Steroids are useful in the short term, and I occasionally will recommend that patients secure treatment from their general practitioner to get the inflammation in their body under control. Nevertheless, they are meant for short-term use and do have side effects. One of the more noticeable side effects is weight gain and water retention. Patients on long-term steroid use tend to have round "baby" faces and put on extra pounds. Prolonged use of steroids can cause soft tissue damage, bone weakness, and osteoporotic changes—which is exactly what we need to avoid—so the use of steroids should be brief and infrequent.

A doctor may prescribe oral steroids or steroid injections such as cortisone or steroid shots. The body produces cortisol, and cortisone is a synthetic reproduction of this natural substance. An injection of these medications maximizes the anti-inflammatory effect more quickly than taking oral medications. The objective of this course of action is to allow the inflammation to decrease, and to allow the patient's body time to heal.

Drugs are never a long-term solution. The body's ability to adapt means that many drugs are less effective over time. The body compensates and begins to create the inflammation again, which is why an increased number of drugs or more powerful drugs must be prescribed. Eventually there is a limit to this course of treatment.

## *Injections*

INJECTIONS MAY BE performed for back or neck pain. If there is any relief, it is often short-lived. Sometimes the injections provide no relief, depending on many factors and a patient's history. There are varying types of injections, and the most prevalent types include epidural, selective nerve root block (SNRB), facet joint block, facet rhizotomy, and sacroiliac joint block.

Epidurals are routinely used to relieve back or neck pain temporarily. The medication, which usually contains an anti-inflammatory to reduce inflammation, is injected directly into the epidural space, which surrounds the spinal cord and contains lymphatics, nerves, and spinal fluid.

The SNRB is a diagnostic procedure performed to determine which spinal nerve root is origin of the pain, in an attempt to gain therapeutic pain relief from inflammation at that nerve root. The SNRB is also performed for the facet joint and sacroiliac joint, but again the results, if any, are short-term and therapeutic.

Each progressive injection may be less effective. This will vary with each patient. Initially, the injections may be beneficial in blocking the pain or decreasing the inflammation, but in the end, these do not do help a patient heal. It buys time, but it is not a cure for the condition. Patients who have had these injections often have said it acted much like a band-aid. They had pain relief for a week or a few months, at best. Inevitably, their pain returned.

One concern about the continued use of pain medications and anti-inflammatories is that these simply mask the pain. Without pain, the patient may continue to perform certain activities or movements that could cause damage to the injured area. The injured area could experience significant degeneration from repetitive injury and from the continued use of steroids. According to one school of thought, if you continue to exercise a joint that is not moving correctly, it may accelerate degeneration of the injured joint by up to 30%.

A more aggressive treatment is facet rhizotomy injection. If a patient had some temporary relief with a series of facet block injections, then a procedure may be performed in which a needle with a probe is inserted near the nerves around the facet joint of the spine. The probe, heated by radio waves, is applied to the sensory nerve related to the facet joint. In theory, this kills the nerve to the joint capsule, which stops pain signals from going to the brain. This technique, also called a nerve ablation, burns and destroys the nerves. This may cause increased pain later.

## *Physical Therapy*

PHYSICAL THERAPY (PT) is the use of designed exercises and equipment to rehabilitate an injury. Physical therapy is often used in conjunction with medication and injections for neck and back pain. The goal of physical therapy is to help extend a patient's range of motion, strengthen muscles, decrease pain, and resume normal activities. Physical therapists educate and instruct the patient on how to work, lift, and move without further injury. Again, many patients who have severe disc conditions end up frustrated because physical therapy rarely changes function enough to correct a problem for the long term, or to avoid surgery.

When an exercise program is prescribed, usually one of two things happens: either pain increases, or any relief is short-lived. Severe pain can limit the ability to bend, stretch, and move. While physical therapy is valuable for treating a serious traumatic injury or a surgical procedure that has damaged muscle that needs to be strengthened, it is my opinion that physical therapy is not as effective for disc-related conditions. In fact, it may cause an exacerbation of the condition. Many of my patients, who were referred to physical therapy, complained that after physical therapy, their symptoms were worse.

## *Acupuncture and Holistic Remedies, or Complementary and Alternative Medical Therapies*

COMPLEMENTARY AND ALTERNATIVE medicine (CAM) is a group of diverse medical and healthcare systems, practices, and products. CAM is generally not thought of as a part of mainstream medicine. At least 38% of adults in the United States use CAM therapies, according to National Center of Complementary Medicine. The following are only a few of the common CAM therapies.

Acupuncture has been one of the principal forms of treatment in traditional Chinese medicine, and it has been practiced for more than 5,000 years. The perspective from which an acupuncturist views health and sickness is the concept of balanced energy.

Acupuncture treatment consists of placing very thin stainless steel needles into the skin of the patient at specific locations—meridian points—that correspond to certain parts of the body associated with energy channels. The goal of acupuncture is to balance the body's chi, or life force. This treatment has been used for thousands of years for a range of problems, including pain. While it can help on a temporary basis, it is not a long-term treatment for pain associated with spinal disc conditions.

In the DRS Protocol™, I provide a homeopathic remedy, Formula 303, to most patients. Homeopathy and homeopathic remedies began in the 18th century, as a gentle alternative treatment to the other harsh forms of medicine that were available. The basis of homeopathy is that substances that produce symptoms of illness will, when given in diluted quantities, stimulate the body's immune system and healing processes.

Formula 303 is a natural muscle relaxant and works well as a tension reliever. Dee Cee Laboratories® has manufactured this formula for over 45 years. Formula 303 is excellent for insomnia, tension, temporomandibular joint (TMJ) pain, back spasm, neck spasm, anxiety, and stress (because being in pain is stressful). This all-natural muscle relaxant can be used for treating a wide range of pain symptoms, and is a safe alternative to prescription drugs. It is non-habit-forming and is effective for pain relief, and is an important part of the DRS Protocol™. Dee Cee Laboratories® is a well-established company with an impeccable reputation. Their products are manufactured under Good Manufacturing Practices (GMPs).

With the DRS Protocol™, all of my patients receive instruction in visualization or guided imagery. Guided imagery is the concept of the mind and body being interconnected and influencing each other. Clinical studies have shown that imagery, or visualization, can affect the physiological responses of the heart, respiratory system, immune functions, cellular growth, pain, relaxation, and sleep.

Homeopathic and guided imagery are often beyond what is offered in a traditional clinical setting. Medical doctors offer a wide array of surgical and diagnostic procedures, but set aside the natural healing ideas.

# Traditional Surgical Interventions and Diagnostic Procedures

THERE ARE TWO different categories of surgical procedures: diagnostic and intervention. Diagnostics include such procedures as a discogram, which is a diagnostic procedure performed prior to a surgical procedure. It is performed to determine definitively which disc is causing the pain and if fusion is required. During this procedure, the doctor slides a needle through the body (through the abdomen if the problem is in the lumbar region) while the patient is awake, though usually sedated. A sterile, saline solution with a radiologic dye is injected into the disc, and the pain response recorded (a positive finding is the re-creation of the actual pain previously reported by the patient). Guided fluoroscopic images (moving X-rays) are made, and the damaged disc is shown on film during the procedure.

Discograms are extremely painful, and someone needs to drive the patient home afterward. It may cause nerve damage in the disc, and it accelerates degeneration of the disc. I believe that a thorough examination and a medical history, along an X-ray or MRI, will give the same information, in most cases.

A myelogram is an X-ray study in which dye is injected into the cerebrospinal fluid, and then the patient is X-rayed to see if there is pressure on the nerves of the spinal cord coming from the disc. This study is important because during the study, the patient's head and torso are raised to a 45° angle. The body, at this angle, puts pressure on the disc, and this shows how the disc might appear in a weight-bearing situation. One serious side effect of the procedure can be arachnoiditis, which is an irritation of the tissue covering the spinal cord, causing severe, long-term pain.

Should the patient opt for surgical intervention, there are also different methods for surgery, depending on the surgeon's specialization and the patient's condition. A discectomy is a procedure to shave off the bulging portion of the disc. Unfortunately, the disc often becomes weaker in the area where the procedure was performed and much more vulnerable to injury. Some doctors perform a discectomy with an arthroscopic laser and the laser will burn off the bulging portion of the disc, while other doctors surgically cut away a portion of the disc.

As with any surgical procedure, there is always the dilemma of the formation of scar tissue. Some doctors inform their patients that scar tissue can form and surgery for its removal may be required. Surgery for the removal of scar tissue may need to be repeated every three to five years. If the removal of scar tissue does not improve their pain, then patients must turn to pain management techniques to help with it.

Another surgical approach is fusion, and there are different surgical procedures that may be used for spinal fusion. They differ in the surgical approach and the instrumentation used. All have advantages and disadvantages. The purpose of fusion is to stop the movement of the vertebrae and immobilize that injured part of the spine, and then allow new grafted bone to grow and stabilize that area into a static position. This can be accomplished by instrumented fusion, which is done by inserting titanium rods on either side of the spine and locking them in place with screws, or by implanting titanium cages. Each has a different surgical approach.

Usually, cages in the lumbar spine are implanted through an incision in the front of the body, and rods are implanted through the back. Each implantation has its risks. Cages have a higher risk of non-fusion and of causing bleeding. For males, there is a chance of retrograde ejaculation because of potential damage to nerves. Each type of fusion can be partnered with bone implants: cadaver bone (harvested from a cadaver), synthetic bone, or bone from the patient's own donation. However, donations can have relatively high risk of complication such as chronic pain after surgery, infection, and pelvic fractures, all associated with the area of the bone harvest.

It can take months—up to 12 months in some cases—for the surgery to heal and stabilize. The problem with spinal fusions is they do not reliably provide long-term positive outcomes, and the patient may be free of pain for only two to three years, if ever. When a fusion is completed, the vertebrae directly above and below the fusion tend to experience accelerated degeneration and are likely to cause a future problem, requiring an additional surgery to fuse the adjacent vertebral levels. A successful fusion is judged on whether it eliminates movement at the fused level—not whether the surgery has reduced pain.

Many researchers conclude there is not sufficient evidence to show that lumbar fusions provide greater improvement for back pain than alternative conservative treatment techniques, such as back education, cognitive behavioral therapy, physical therapy, exercise, weight reduction, and alternative therapies. The DRS Protocol™ can improve pain from the disc problem of the level above and below the fused portion of the spine, but nothing can be done to change the fused area. Despite the uncertainty of fusions, lumbar fusions increased nearly four-fold between 1992 and 2003.

Another surgical procedure for degenerative disc disease is disc replacement, and there are several types of implants. Simply explained, this surgery involves removing the disc and replacing it with an artificial implant. These procedures are performed primarily on the lumbar spine. Many surgeons are reluctant to perform disc replacements because they are not entirely proven, there is no long-term relief (many candidates are young people), and the procedure is controversial. One frequent question from many of my patients is, "Can't a bad disc just be replaced with a good one?" Disc replacement is still in clinical trials, and there is no understanding on how they will work in the long term. In my opinion, this is a very radical procedure, and I believe patients should steer clear of it. Disc replacement patients cannot be treated with the DRS Protocol™ or spinal decompression.

Decompressive laminectomy is a surgical procedure that removes a piece of the bony arch, or lamina, on the dorsal surface of a vertebra. It is much like lifting the top off a tunnel. A portion of the vertebra is lifted off exposing the spinal cord to relieve pressure on the spinal cord and nerves.

With age, discs begin to degenerate, and the vertebrae in the spine become much closer to each other, which can result in bone spurs and ligamentum flavum in hypertrophy (a condition where the spinal canal narrows, causing pressure on the nerves). These cause the spinal canal and the foramina to narrow, which may pinch the spinal nerves. Different studies report different success rates, and even surgeons' success rates will differ. Laminectomies were performed more routinely in the past. However, they are still being done.

Patients who have had any of these previous surgeries and are still in pain can have good results with the DRS Protocol™, with the exception of those who have had a disc replacement.

Patients who have disc surgery have a variance in outcomes, with most falling into the areas described below. Outcomes may also be influenced by age, diagnosis, and other health conditions.

1.  **Little or no improvement:** According to a study in the June 15, 2005 issue of Spine, 40% of patients who undergo spinal surgery have little or no improvement. Although pain might change from a sharp pain to a dull aching pain, surgery really provides no relief. It is common for radiating pain in the leg or arm to be resolved by surgery, but a patient may continue to experience a considerable amount of back or neck pain.

2.  **Moderate improvement:** Another 20% saw moderate improvement while 40% had improvement one year post-surgery. Of course, there are patients who will have excellent results, though it is not very common. Even those who initially show improvement will statistically be more likely to experience problems within a few years. Discovery Times TV reported in an exposé in 2005 that back surgery failure is estimated to be as high as 78% in the United States due to underreporting of ongoing problems suffered by patients, and the overuse of surgery as a cure for pain. This means that surgery is routinely recommended for patients who have other health conditions that will interfere with their ability to have a successful outcome, so the results can be very disappointing.

3.  **Worse pain following surgery:** This is very common, as often the surgery injures other tissue and causes scar tissue to form that creates more pain.

4.  **Permanent damage, numbness, muscle weakness, or muscle atrophy:** Any of these outcomes is possible. When the body is cut open, damage can be done to vital structures within the spine, which can cause permanent damage and disability.

5.  **All other risks inherent in surgery:** Other risks include infection and even death.

Even when patients feel their surgery has had a good outcome because they initially feel better, they do not realize how much weaker their spine is after surgery. Jack's story is a sad, yet strong example of this point. He had previously had a discectomy, the surgical removal of part or all of a vertebral disc that has herniated. Jack was pleased with the outcome at that point. Two weeks later, as he was returning for his post-surgical follow-up examination, he had an unfortunate experience. He was on the elevator and it stopped just a few inches above the floor level, and Jack did not notice. As he walked off the elevator, he stepped down hard and jolted his back. He reherniated the same disc, right there in the medical building.

Jack came to me for treatment with the DRS Protocol™ because he absolutely was not going through surgery again. Surgery is a traumatic procedure for any part of the body, let alone the spine. He felt that if his spine was that weak after the first surgery, then he did not want to go through it again and have the risk of continuing pain.

Even if a patient has failed back or neck surgery and is experiencing post-surgery pain, he or she can begin DRS Protocol™. The waiting period is only four to six weeks. However, if a patient has had spinal fusion, where bones and instrumentation were implanted, the required wait is at least six to eight months. This allows time for the bone and surrounding tissue to heal completely and become as stable as possible. It is important to remember that the fused level of the patient's spine will not be able to be treated. However, the adjacent levels above and below the fusion can be treated with the DRS Protocol™. Patient welfare and a good outcome are paramount to me.

# Spinal Cord Stimulators

PATIENTS STILL EXPERIENCING post-surgical pain because of failed surgery for a disc condition will often have to move into a pain management program. Ultimately, pain pumps and spinal cord stimulators are prescribed in an attempt to maintain their pain at a livable level. The pain pump is a small device implanted under the skin and intermittently injects medication directly into the spinal cord.

Spinal cord stimulators are another alternative for control of pain from failed back surgeries, chronic pain, and nerve damage. A small wire or lead, which connects to a power source, is implanted surgically in the spinal cord. Electrical signals are transmitted through the lead to the spinal cord or to specific nerves to block pain signals from reaching the brain.

Some stimulators use a remote control to turn the current off or on and to adjust intensity. There are two types: one is an implanted unit that uses a pulse generator and a non-rechargeable battery that is replaced over time. The second system employs radio frequencies, and it uses a transmitter with an antenna, which is much like a cell phone, and a receiver, and is implanted in the body. The patient has to have had a successful trial period with the spinal cord stimulator before a permanent stimulator is implanted.

Pain is the body's means of communicating there is a problem. Spinal cord stimulation interferes with nerve transmission of pain. It does not address the underlying problem. Possible risks of spinal cord stimulations include hardware failure and scar tissue (fibrosis) formation around the electrode, which may increase pain and reduces the effectiveness of the stimulator. The patient may have pain that gradually moves beyond the reach of the nerve stimulator, rendering it useless. In addition, the patient's body may compensate, and the stimulator could become less effective.

Since the device is a piece of hardware, this allows for the possibility of the hardware breaking. Additional surgery may be necessary to replace the device because of complications, failures, or lead migration and breakage.

The implantation of a foreign object in the body has the risk of causing infection in the spine. Spinal cord stimulators or pain pumps can cause the leakage of spinal fluid and disabling headaches. The increased stimulation from spinal cord stimulators may also cause bladder problems.

Treatment success with spinal cord stimulators is influenced by the cause of pain, if there has been a previous back surgery, and the amount of time that has passed since the surgery. The longer the time since a first surgery, the less likely that spinal cord stimulation will overpower the pain signals that have developed. Often, when a spinal stimulator stops working, it is just left inside the patient. It is not removed or replaced.

When I consult with a patient who has a working spinal cord stimulator, I do not treat the area where the stimulator is implanted. If the patient's implant is not working, then it is preferable to have the stimulator removed before beginning treatment with the DRS Protocol™. There are many reasons to be cautious with spinal cord stimulators. The primary reason is the leads can be pulled out of place with spinal decompression treatment or chiropractic manipulation.

# Chiropractic Care and Spinal Decompression

CHIROPRACTIC, BY DEFINITION of the American Chiropractic Association, is a healthcare profession that focuses on disorders of the musculoskeletal system and the nervous system, and the effects these disorders have on overall health. Chiropractic care is used most often to treat neuromusculoskeletal complaints, including back pain, neck pain, headaches, and pain in the joints of the arms or legs. Chiropractors perform spinal manipulation or spinal adjustments in order to restore function of the nervous system and the spine, which alleviates the pressure on the nerves, muscle tightness, pain, and allows the tissue to heal. Spinal manipulation does not hurt. However, occasionally a patient may experience mild soreness, much like after working out for the first time. Doctors of Chiropractic do not prescribe drugs or perform surgery.

Traditional chiropractic care is very effective in the conservative care and management of back and neck pain and disc-related conditions. However, there is a level of severity of a disc condition that surpasses the effectiveness of treatment with chiropractic care.

The DRS Protocol™ uses spinal decompression, specific chiropractic manipulation, nutrition, and exercise to provide a more encompassing treatment and management protocol for chronic and severe disc conditions. A patient with a disc condition may have previously responded to chiropractic care, but as the condition progressively worsens, there may be a limit to what chiropractic treatment can do for continued improvement. For these patients, I treat with the DRS Protocol™ and improvement is seen quickly. Naturally, each patient progresses according to the diagnosis, lifestyle, habits, and other health factors.

Both chiropractic and spinal decompression are gentle, noninvasive and are intended to restore normal function to the body. They work well together, and allow the body to heal naturally.

Spinal decompression, which is safe, noninvasive, and pain-free, employs a computerized distractive force over a logarithmic curve that can override the body's natural defense mechanism of tightening the muscles in response to external pulling. This logarithmic curve allows the application of specific amounts of force to be applied to the spine directly at the level of the disc injury, either of the lumbar or cervical spine. The level of the spine to be treated is controlled by the angle at which the force is applied to the spine.

Spinal decompression employs a computerized program with patient-specific parameters, angles, and weight-of-pull that is customized and can be retained in the software for each individual. Most importantly, spinal decompression uses the application of ramping, which slowly introduces axial force to the spine. This creates a wider spacing of the vertebral discs, which in turn, creates a negative internal disc pressure (decompression). The bulging material from the disc will retract back into the disc and off the spinal cord and nerves.

The DRS Protocol™ is a successful system of treatment elements: spinal decompression, chiropractic care, and other elements that facilitate healing. I am offering my patients a choice that is a successful alternative to surgery.

The protocol meets a full range of patient needs and helps to facilitate healing. Patients can expect outcomes in the following categories:

1.  **High percentage of improvement or dramatic improvement:** There is frequently 100% improvement, which means the patient is back to a normal life and pain free.

2.  **Large percentage improvement with decreased pain and less muscle spasm:** Patients may have more strength but will not be completely back to the way they were pre-injury. However, patients have achieved substantial improvement and will return to a normal, full lifestyle. The patient who has had long-standing degenerative disc disease pain may now only notice pain when the area is aggravated by a specific activity.

3.  **Patient responds well to treatment and has had pain for so long that the improvement is life altering, although the condition is not totally resolved:** The patient who has had long-standing degenerative pain may still be limited in certain activities, but will be largely improved.

4.  **Patient has improvement in some areas, but not all:** There is improvement in some areas of complaint, but the results are not dramatic. This category represents a small percentage of all patients.

Nowhere in the list does death or spinal cord damage appear, nor do any other inherent risks of surgery appear or apply to the DRS Protocol™. This particular point alone makes a particularly convincing reason to research conservative, noninvasive care.

# CHAPTER 6

*Nutrition and Fitness*

# CHAPTER SIX

## *Nutrition and Fitness*

W hen dealing with patients experiencing chronic pain, there are many questions that need to be asked, and some of those involve a topic that many people try to avoid: diet. A little known fact for patients who experience pain is that there are some things they can do nutritionally to help themselves decrease inflammation and, as a result, experience less pain.

There are many schools of thought regarding nutrition—far too many to cover here. I am primarily focusing on some standard ideas, and I will leave the debate about the perfect diet to another book. After all, this is not about the perfect diet, this is about improvement.

When a new patient is evaluated, a history of medications, supplements, over-the-counter pain relievers, and other remedies is compiled. Information is gathered about overall nutritional habits. In certain cases, when a patient has had a severe long-term problem, the assessment must go deeper. I need to look into the regular dietary habits to determine how much protein, fats, and carbohydrates are consumed. Many doctors do not relate a disc condition to the subject of nutrition and digestion, but there is a compelling reason for this line of inquiry. Many back and neck problems, along with headaches, can be related to systemic inflammation caused by diet, a lifestyle of alcohol and tobacco use, and the inability to absorb or digest nutrients.

Patients who have continuing problems of indigestion, constipation, or diarrhea rarely think of these as serious. However, these are symptoms of underlying problems. Usually, these problems do not send people to the doctor before serious complications begin, and they commonly use over-the-counter (OTC) products to deal with them.

Using these products, in addition to pain relievers, becomes a means of continuing to self-medicate. Some offer relief, but they cannot correct conditions that have been disguised for years. A good example of an OTC remedy is an antacid, which may interact with medicines. Many medications warn against the use of antacids. Additionally, some antacids will contain aluminum or a large amount of sodium, and they may create a laxative effect or cause constipation.

## Cause and Effect

SOME FOODS WILL directly contribute to inflammation as well as the pain from inflammation. This not only slows the patient's response to care but can also serve to discourage the patient. The food we eat—or do not eat—affects how our bodies function. We need a variety of foods to be able to heal properly and quickly. Some patients who have a greater difficulty with healing are those with dietary restrictions or poor diets in general.

While you may think that this does not apply to you, prepackaged food, especially junk food, has been through extensive processing that destroys its nutritional value. Highly refined products such as white flour, white sugar, and white rice are stripped of most nutritional content. Processing will remove much of the flavor and change the appearance of food. This problem is fixed by adding artificial flavors and colors. Some flavorings are actually chemicals and are used because they are cheaper than real flavors. Because food needs to be shipped long distances and have a long shelf life, preservatives are added. Hormones and antibiotics are added to beef, chicken, and milk sold to the public, and the effects of these on the human body have hardly been considered. Preservatives and pesticides can have cumulative and detrimental effects on our bodies, and processed foods lose most of their vitamins, minerals, enzymes during the preservation process.

## *Stay Close to Nature*

WHOLE FOODS THAT are closest to their natural form are best for our bodies. They are not overly processed or adulterated with excess of salt, sugar, additives, and fat. Foods that supply most nutrients are grains, fish, fruit, and vegetables. In today's hurried world, people eat a diet of fast food, junk food, and prepackaged food, without realizing that they are inhibiting their body's ability to heal and increasing inflammation.

Most do not understand what nutrients the body needs. Popular diets may convince them that certain elements of foods are "bad," leading them to avoid those items. Many different foods are necessary for good health. I have listed a few of the most essential in this chapter. While this is by no means a complete list, it will give you an idea of how a lack of these items affects your body and why it is important to be educated about proper nutrition.

# A Tale of Two Carbs

RESEARCH IS INCREASINGLY turning attention to the consequences of poor and inadequate digestion as the source of chronic degenerative problems such as myofibrosis and arthritis.

As with all foods, there are desirable elements and less desirable elements. Contrary to popular belief, carbohydrates are not an enemy. There are good carbohydrates and bad carbohydrates. Carbohydrates are a main source of energy for our bodies. There are three kinds of carbohydrates: fiber, sugars, and starches. The body will use some carbohydrates for immediate energy, while converting others to fat to use later.

Carbohydrates have gotten a bad rap in the news and in the minds of the general population because of the easy availability of simple carbohydrates. Simple carbohydrates are abundant in fast food, junk food, and a whole variety of "foods" that have nothing in common with the food humans consumed prior to the last 50 years. These include potato chips, sodas, lattes, and pretty much anything found in the "snack" aisle of the grocery store.

Many diet programs urge the reduction or even elimination of carbohydrates from the diet. However, carbohydrates are used by the body exclusively for energy. A diet that excludes carbohydrates can produce side effects such as weakness, brain fog, constipation, and stiffness in the joints. Complex carbohydrates are actually a necessary part of a balanced diet. They are very important in the production of energy, and they are found in the following foods:

- wheat germ
- bran
- barley
- maize

- buckwheat
- cornmeal
- oatmeal
- brown rice
- pasta
- whole grain breads
- muesli
- root vegetables, such as potatoes and yams
- squash
- peas
- lentils
- corn

THESE FOODS ARE good sources of complex carbohydrates, and when consumed in as close to a natural state as possible; they are wonderful sources of energy for the body. This is not a complete list of complex carbohydrates, just a good starting point. Eating foods in their simplest, organic form will provide the most benefits.

When treating disc-related conditions, a main objective is to reduce inflammation, so the nerves and tissue can recover. Simple carbohydrates interfere with that process. Simple carbohydrates not only contribute to weight gain and are empty calories, but some can contribute to the inflammatory process of the body, and that can slow healing which makes the patient less responsive to care.

## *Protein*

PROTEIN FROM ANIMAL sources has been shunned by those who espouse a vegetarian philosophy. Normal sources of protein in a regular diet include red meat, poultry, fish, and eggs. Protein is also found in plant products, dairy, legumes, nuts, and seeds. These foods should be part of a well-rounded diet. Skin, bones, muscles, and organs contain protein. Protein is in the blood, hormones, and enzymes. The body needs a little bit of everything to be healthy. A diet low in protein is also often deficient in iron, zinc, thiamin, and vitamin B6. Protein is a major building block in the amino acids of the body and plays a major role in cellular function. Glucose is also obtained from protein. It is absorbed more slowly into the bloodstream, and it does not cause a rapid increase in blood sugar. Unlike glucose, the body does not store much protein, and if it becomes deficient in protein, this will cause the muscle to break down, much in the same manner as when people starve.

While vegetarians and vegans avoid meat, they still need protein for their bodies to function correctly. Protein is an essential building block that helps create cells and helps the healing process. While almost all vegetarian and vegan diet programs stress the need to seek sources of protein other than animal sources, it can be challenging to consume enough protein. Many patients I treat are vegetarians, and some of them tend to be protein-deficient. Many vegetarians eat soy-based products and soybeans. While these are high in protein, they also include phytoestrogens, which can have unintended effects—especially in post-menopausal women, where they have been shown to contribute to bone loss and increase the risk of vertebral fractures. In children, phytoestrogens can cause early menses and other developmental changes.

Even if you choose not to include soy products in your diet, there are other natural sources of protein, such as nuts and sweet potatoes. Below is a partial list (the amounts are for one-cup portions) and a comparison with the amounts of protein found in examples of meat sources:

## Non-meat sources

- lentils (18 grams of protein)
- black beans (15 grams)
- kidney beans (13 grams)
- chickpeas (12 grams)
- vegetarian baked beans (12 grams)
- pinto beans (12 grams)
- black-eyed peas (11 grams)
- peas (9 grams)
- spinach (5 grams)
- broccoli (4 grams)

## Meat sources

- 4 ounces chicken breast (35 grams of protein)
- 3 ounces beef (26 grams)
- 3 ounces turkey (25 grams)
- 3 ounces salmon (23 grams)

THESE ARE A few examples of protein sources. I would encourage anyone to research various sources of protein and to make certain to consume enough to support their body and maintain good health.

## Fat

FATS ARE NOT automatically the enemy. They help the body absorb vitamins, maintain the structure and function of cells, and help maintain the immune system. Fats provide the energy and help create an energy reserve. Fats also help maintain a consistent body temperature. They are also involved in the production and regulation of steroids within the body.

"Fat is bad," has become a popular mantra for the food industry over the past couple of decades. Food products now tout reduced fat, low fat, or no fat. In our quest to control weight and improve health, marketers have learned that by producing and promoting products with less fat, they increase sales. However, fat is an essential element in constructing and maintaining cell membrane, and fat aids the body in absorbing essential vitamins. Without enough of the right kind of fat, cells cannot function as well, and this includes the cells of the nervous system, which includes the spinal cord. The right kind of fat is required for good health.

What is the right kind of fat? Good fats are the omega-3 fatty acids. Some easy to find sources of omega-3 fatty acids are walnuts, flaxseed, beans, fish, olive oil, squash, and cold-water fish. Omega-3 fats help limit inflammation by producing certain chemicals in the body that will aid in controlling inflammation. These chemicals will reduce (or, more correctly, inhibit) inflammation.

Fats to avoid include any hydrogenated fats, such as saturated and trans fats, and oils derived from corn or cottonseed. While eating products light in fat is not a bad course of action, especially if you trying to watch your weight, you have to be aware that some fat is required for health. Studies now show that even butter in moderate amounts is healthy, although using olive oil would be preferred.

One item of note when discussing fat is cholesterol. Cholesterol cannot dissolve in the blood. It has to be transported to and from the cells by carriers called lipoproteins. There are two types of cholesterol. Low-density lipoprotein, or LDL, is known as "bad" cholesterol. High-density lipoprotein, or HDL, is known as "good" cholesterol. These two types of lipids, along with triglycerides and Lp(a) cholesterol, make up your total cholesterol count, which can be determined through a standard blood test.

When too much LDL cholesterol is in the blood, it can build up on the walls of the arteries and form plaque—a hard deposit that can narrow the arteries and make them less flexible—which is a condition known as atherosclerosis. If a clot forms and blocks a narrowed artery, a heart attack or stroke can result.

About one-fourth to one-third of blood cholesterol is carried by high-density lipoprotein (HDL). HDL cholesterol is known as "good" cholesterol because high levels seem to protect against heart attack, while low levels increase the risk of heart disease. Medical experts think that HDL carries cholesterol away from the arteries and back to the liver, where it is passed from the body. Some experts believe that HDL removes excess cholesterol from arterial plaque, slowing its buildup.

Triglyceride is a form of fat made in the body. The causes of elevated triglycerides can include obesity, physical inactivity, smoking, excess alcohol consumption, and a diet very high in carbohydrates (60% or more of total calories). People with high triglycerides often have a high total cholesterol level, including a high LDL level and a low HDL level. Many people with heart disease or diabetes also have high triglyceride levels.

I am often asked about specific types of synthetic fats, such as margarine, which was promoted as heart-healthy for years. However, margarine contains large amounts of trans fats from hydrogenated oils. My stance is that if it does not occur in nature or by pressing something natural, such as olives or coconut, then you should probably not eat it. Eat organically or as close to the natural source as possible.

# Anti-Inflammatory Foods

MANY GOOD FOOD choices will help decrease pain from inflammation:

## Vegetables

- bok choy
- broccoli
- brussels sprouts
- cabbage
- cauliflower
- chard
- collards
- garlic
- green beans
- green onions/spring onions
- kale
- leeks
- olives
- spinach
- sweet potatoes

## Fruits

- apples
- avocados
- black currants
- blueberries
- kiwi fruit
- lemons
- limes

- oranges
- papaya
- pineapple (fresh)
- raspberries
- rhubarb
- strawberries
- cherries

## *Protein*

- beef (lean organic)
- chicken breast (skinless, boneless, and organic)
- oysters
- rainbow trout
- salmon
- snapper
- striped bass
- whitefish

## *Oils*

- avocado
- coconut
- olive

THERE IS SOME preliminary indication that plants in the night-shade family can increase inflammation in the body. These plants include tomatoes, eggplant, peppers, and potatoes. These plants contain a substance called solanine, which may increase inflammation and pain in certain people. The best course of action is to eliminate this category from the diet for two weeks, and then reintroduce it to see if pain and inflammation increases.

# *Hydration*

FEW PEOPLE DRINK enough water. I do not mean liquid. Many people drink coffee, sodas, tea, or other drinks all day, but they do not drink enough water. The problem is compounded by the fact that many of these other drinks can have adverse effects on a person's health.

Our bodies are made up of 70% water, and water is necessary for the body to function. Humans can live without food for literally weeks. Without water, we would last a few days to a week at most. Dehydration compounds any health issue by preventing the cells from getting enough fluid to function properly and by reducing the body's ability to eliminate waste. When the body is dehydrated, cellular waste builds up in the tissue, rather than being carried out of the body via the kidneys.

Proper hydration is critical for recovery for any condition. Not only does it help clear away the results of cellular metabolism (i.e., waste), it is also very important for many other cellular reactions as well. Fluid is important for cellular function.

The majority of my patients I talk with believe they are drinking enough water, but this is rarely the case. A good rule is to drink 8-10, 8-ounce glasses a day, or more when exercising or in a hot environment. That adds up to 64-80 ounces a day. I recommend that a patient fill a pitcher with the amount of water they should drink each day and then drink that amount. They are surprised how much water it really is and quickly realize they are under-hydrating their bodies. The joints of the spine and the discs rely on the hydraulic properties of water and the hydration of the cartilage for proper function as well as the ability to heal.

Many elderly patients may limit their fluid intake because of their own physical problems and limitations, such as arthritis, Alzheimer's, and stroke. The thirst sensation can diminish, and it may be difficult for them to drink enough water. The elderly, or anyone suffering from incontinence, may deliberately limit their fluid intake. All this plays a role in dehydration.

Health issues can be exacerbated by caffeine, which can cause restlessness, anxiety, irritability, tremors, sleeplessness, headaches, gastrointestinal symptoms, and abnormal heart rhythms. In some individuals, caffeine can increase blood pressure. Some people are extra-sensitive to even small amounts of caffeine and can have headaches as a result.

Low back pain can be exacerbated by caffeine. Many people cannot make it through their day without sodas and coffee. These can create inflammation, and they stress the kidneys. Kidney stress/disease can cause low back pain that mimics other conditions. Caffeine, which is a mild diuretic, also can interfere with mineral absorption and utilization. There are also serious side effects from the aspartame in diet drinks and sugar-free products. Aspartame should be avoided!

## *Vitamins and Minerals*

THERE ARE NUMEROUS vitamins and minerals that are essential in helping your body heal. Vitamin C is one of the most well known. It is water-soluble and is not stored in the body. Vitamin C is important in the formation of collagen. Therefore, it is an important part of the spinal disc. It is also an important component of blood vessels, tendons, ligaments, and bone. In addition to the spinal discs, the tissues that most require vitamin C are bone, scar tissue, and blood vessels. These tissues contain a large amount of collagen. Therefore, vitamin C is important in the treatment of disc-related conditions. Vitamin C deficiency can contribute to irregular scar tissue formation, which is not as strong.

It is important to include B vitamins, especially B6 (pyridoxine), which is involved in more bodily functions than any other vitamin. B6 benefits both physical and mental health. It aids in breaking down protein and helps maintain healthy red blood cells, the nervous system, and the immune system. B6 is also a vital part of producing neurotransmitters, the chemicals that allow the brain and nerves to communicate. It also is beneficial for nerve compression conditions and arthritis. In many ways, B6 helps the nerves heal. This has been used for many years as an adjunct to the treatment of carpal tunnel syndrome. All B vitamins are water-soluble and are instrumental in supporting growth, development, and chemical reactions in the body. They are also an important part of turning food into energy. When a person is under stress, it is a good idea to supplement with B vitamins.

I provide vitamins C, B6, and other products, such as Bromelain, to my patients from the exclusively professional products line of Douglas Laboratories, a manufacturer of quality nutritional supplements. For more than 50 years, Douglas Laboratories, a member of the Atrium Innovations, Inc., family of companies, has committed itself to its mission to provide a custom approach to nutrition and wellness. Its standards reflect a dedication to wellness by providing the highest quality nutritional supplements. Douglas Laboratories has the finest reputation and all products are manufactured under Good Manufacturing Practices (GMPs).

A balanced diet that includes grain products, vegetables, and fruits should be adequate to supply all the B vitamins needed. However, since most people do not eat a sufficient amount, there is a definite need to supplement the B vitamins.

I often recommend calcium, the most abundant mineral found in the body, and magnesium, which works in tandem with calcium. Together they play an important role in maintaining healthy bones and a healthy nervous system. People who eat large amounts of processed foods (with most the magnesium is removed) are not getting enough magnesium in their diets.

Calcium makes up 99% of bones and teeth, and it plays major part in maintaining the bones. Calcium and magnesium affect the nervous system and function as natural tranquilizers. They are both sleep aids, in addition to preventing muscle spasms.

It is common for patients who live in pain from disc-related problems to have a heightened sense of pain associated with muscle spasms. In addition to Formula 303, calcium and magnesium help reduce the pain and calm the spasms, which in turn will help patients sleep more comfortably and readily.

Other supplementations can be important in the healing process of the disc and cartilage in general. I have discussed the supplements that I predominantly use in my practice.

It is important to understand that the body uses vitamins and minerals with the help of enzymes. Enzymes in the body are catalysts, and most are a class of protein. The purpose of enzymes is to facilitate chemical reactions, such as the breaking down of protein. This function is dependent on a substance called protease, which is an enzyme that specifically aids in the breaking down of protein.

Enzymes should occur naturally in the food we eat and allow us to break down nutritional substances so they can be fully used by our bodies. Without these enzymes, the nutritional value is lost. It is important to understand that the best source of enzymes is food that is in its natural form, grown in healthy conditions. In order to preserve foods by canning or other methods to allow for shipping and storage, enzymes are destroyed by food processing and manufacturing. Therefore, the more food is processed, the less the body is able to derive proper nutrients. When patients are enzyme-deficient, they frequently suffer from chronic digestive disorders. Because the body has difficulty breaking down food, referred pain may be experienced.

Remember, referred pain is pain that is felt in a different place in the body other than the source. For example, with the gall bladder or heart, pain manifests in another area, such as the left shoulder or arm for the heart, or the right elbow or shoulder for the gall bladder. There is a host of these reflex patterns throughout the body. These are a result of muscle spasm and nerve irritation because there is stress on the body or organ system that corresponds to certain reflex points/patterns. Often, patients who experience chronic degenerative conditions and have these referral patterns will benefit from enzyme therapy.

Enzyme replacement therapy, the art and science of using nutrition to maintain homeostasis and health in the body, was pioneered by a colleague of mine, Dr. Howard Loomis. He is the founder and president of Enzyme Formulations, Inc. Dr. Loomis trains and certifies doctors to evaluate patients through a physical examination process, blood tests, and a 24-hour urinalysis. A patient that I would test is one who is slow to respond to care or has reached a plateau in their progress, or a patient with a very chronic condition and other chronic complaints such as fatigue, headache, and digestive disturbances. These patients may have problems breaking down protein or may be protein-deficient. This type of patient can easily be tested for an underlying nutritional or digestive problem. This problem can be addressed with enzyme replacements, which in many cases easily stabilizes the patient's condition.

I often see patients with chronic lumbar disc conditions, a situation in which their spine or pelvis will never completely stabilize. This type of patient describes the problem as if something in the back or pelvis "just goes out." These patients will benefit from an enzyme, TRCTN. The purpose of TRCTN is to provide a source of vitamins and minerals from protein nutritive herbs combined with enzymes. I have found that this product helps the patient's pelvis stabilize, and I like to call it the "pelvic stabilizer." If the patient's problem is related to spinal nerve damage or irritation and the spine does not stabilize, then the patient should benefit from CMPRS. The purpose of CMPRS is to provide a source of vitamins and minerals from alterative, lymphatic, and diuretic herbs. I refer to this as the "spinal stabilizer." These are a professional line of products from Enzyme Formulations, Inc.

## Herbal Therapies

HERBS ARE DIFFERENT from vitamins. They are derived from plants that are also used in the pharmaceutical industry. It is necessary that your doctor is aware of everything you are taking, even if it is not a prescription. While it may seem that herbs are harmless, there are situations where they could interfere with other medications. For some conditions, they are contraindicated. There can be variations in strength and quality among manufacturers, and for that reason, it is important to do your research on the company providing your herbs and supplements to ensure they are of excellent quality.

## Detrimental Substances

SOME OTHER ELEMENTS that affect patients may include both simple and complex issues, such as excessive coffee or alcohol intake. A patient may also have a slower response to care due to poor nutrition. It is well understood that both smoking and excessive alcohol consumption are detrimental to our health. Nicotine is a powerful drug that leeches minerals such as calcium from bone and decreases blood supply.

Alcohol should never be used as a means of self-medicating for chronic pain. Alcohol may act as a short-term muscle relaxant but provides no therapeutic effect and can adversely affect health and limit healing. Over time, other health problems may develop, such as high blood pressure, along with liver and digestive problems. Alcohol is a depressant, and those who abuse it can develop both physical and emotional dependency.

## *Physical Activity*

WHEN IT COMES to good health, movement is life. Staying fit is very important for our bodies, and this is especially true about the spine. It is important to maintain flexibility and range of motion, especially to heal after an injury or to decrease the effects of a degenerative disease.

One of the simplest and best ways to exercise is to walk. Walking strengthens the spine and maintains good overall health. I frequently recommend that patients lift some light weights to create resistance and rebuild muscles that may have atrophied from lack of use during an injury. You do not have to purchase expensive weights. Exercise bands or even cans of vegetables provide enough resistance to help the spine. Stretching is very important as the muscles tend to spasm, which causes decreased blood flow. Stretching lengthens these muscles again, facilitating free blood flow and increased oxygen levels.

Patients ask if they should focus on low-impact or high-impact exercise to get back into shape after a disc-related problem. The best avenue is to begin slowly. One of the biggest mistakes is to attempt to return to the level of exercise prior to the injury. When returning to exercise, it must begin slowly and moderately, so as to avoid re-injury. Consistent exercise and gradually working up to the level of exercise previously enjoyed is important.

I had a patient in his early 40s, who was responding well to the DRS Protocol™, and he had achieved an 80% sustained improvement, after just a few weeks of care. Suddenly, he stopped making progress and even took a step back in improvement. We talked several times about what might be the problem. After an additional two weeks of treatment and re-evaluation, he finally confessed he had started running again. His goal was to run in a race that was a month away. I strongly advised him to allow his spine to heal first, but he refused. Because he refused to comply with his treatment plan, I had to release him from care. The patient was not able to complete the run, and he ended up having a spinal fusion. He did not run that year or any time thereafter, due to complications from his spinal fusion. This story illustrates that patience and focus are required to heal fully. The good from treatment can be undone if the body is not allowed sufficient time to recover.

Early in the treatment with the DRS Protocol™, specific exercises such as running and weightlifting must be avoided, although this does not mean that the patient will never be able to resume these activities. It is important to avoid certain exercises that increase the disc pressure and cause re-injury of the disc.

One area of concern is exercise equipment. There is a variety of equipment including stationary bicycles, stair climbers, treadmills, and elliptical trainers. Riding a recumbent bicycle is great exercise when a patient is ready. However, equipment such as ellipticals may put an unnatural stress on the spine and exacerbate a condition. It is better to choose exercise equipment that will not alter the normal gait or biomechanics.

The benefits of exercising in the water are many. Aquatic exercise, such as swimming, improves cardiovascular fitness, endurance, and overall strength. Aquatic exercise gives the benefit of a non-weight bearing environment and reduces the likelihood of injury. Exercise balls are also popular and can help with balance and increasing the strength of core abdominal muscles. While using exercise balls is not for everyone, they are good for some patients. Simply balancing in a sitting position each day can help greatly. I use exercise balls in my practice because I have seen a great benefit for my patients who have used them.

Every patient is different, so I recommend various exercises and methods according to the needs and recovery of each individual. Once recovered, I encourage my patients to exercise regularly to keep their bodies in optimal shape to avoid another injury. I also instruct my patients to continue the specific back or neck exercises they were given during the course of their treatment.

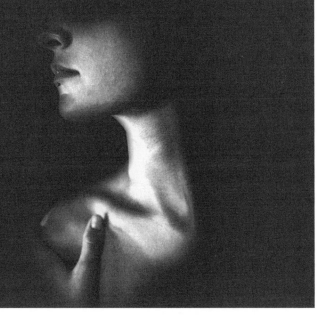

# CHAPTER 7

*Healing Starts in the Mind*

# CHAPTER SEVEN

## *Healing Starts in the Mind*

When I was in chiropractic college, professors would often discuss the philosophy of treating the whole person and not just the physical body. The role of the mind in healthcare has been observed for years, and there are competing schools of thought that are complex and multifaceted. There is a mind-body-spirit connection that is real and powerful. I know when I enlist my patients' minds in their own care, they respond faster.

We have all heard of people who were living normal, seemingly healthy lives, and suddenly they were diagnosed with a serious disease. Within a short time, some patients succumb to their diagnosis. The fascinating psychological aspect of this is that what happens next may depend upon that person's perspective of the disease and the individual's beliefs. I believe the diagnosis, in many cases, can be as terminal as the disease. When a patient allows the fear of the disease into thought, then the disease process is given the full strength and beliefs of the mind, and it is allowed to flourish. With some, this almost acts as a death sentence. On the positive side, studies show that cancer patients who have positive attitudes toward their disease have higher survival rates. Evidence suggests that what matters is the attitude toward the disease. This shows there are benefits to adopting a survivor attitude.

There are surgeons who will not operate on a patient if that patient is too mentally depressed or is convinced that the outcome will be less than favorable. When dealing with the human body, it important to remember is that it is not "just a body." There is also a "being," and the "being" brings with it its own memories, thoughts and beliefs. Those will affect the way that "being," responds to any type of care for any type problem.

The whole idea of a mind-body connection is that the attitude of the patient has a positive effect on a patient's overall health, recovery, and outcome. Guided imagery is used to work with and through this mind-body connection to aid in the healing process. Emotions can influence the immune system in either a positive or a negative way, and patients have the ability to choose, merely by their attitude.

It is important to understand the emotional, psychological, and mental factors that play into the healing of the patient. When I am dealing with a patient, I take all of this into consideration. It is much easier to help a patient who believes health is possible. Conversely, it is much harder to help someone who does not believe help is possible, or is convinced that the situation is hopeless.

An area I focus on when treating someone is to teach the patient to perform visualization exercises or guided imagery for healing. I believe if the patient can see it and believe it, it is more likely to happen. There is also the verse from Proverbs: "As a man thinketh so is he." I believe this is most accurate.

The connection between a patient's state of mind and the ability to heal cannot be ignored. The mind is very powerful, and it can alter the way the body functions. With visualization exercises, the patient is removing any barriers that may be present in the way of thoughts and beliefs. In essence, the whole patient is being treated, not just the physical malady. It does not matter how great a treatment is, if the mind is not convinced about potential improvement, then no treatment will produce optimal results. For this reason, it is essential to recruit the mind into the equation.

I ask patients to visualize their lives without pain. I ask them to think about what they want to do and where they want to go, and to imagine and visualize all those little activities that will suddenly be easy again—things such as getting in and out of a vehicle, being able to work all day, going to the grocery store or to the mall, or preparing a meal. This is especially important if a patient has been in pain for an extended period of time, as the pain takes away all focus, and it is difficult for a patient to even imagine being without it.

I also ask patients to imagine their bodies repairing the injured area. We look at illustrations of healthy vertebrae and discs, and then ask that they imagine healing, the inflammation disappearing, and their nerves being relieved from pressure. Patients are to do this for a few moments each treatment and again at home. It is also important for patients to understand that they must do these visualization exercises each day.

Professional sports teams, Olympic athletes, and NASA have used visualization for years. What the mind can see, the body can achieve, and this same idea can be applied to healing. I was introduced to the idea of visualization through sports as a child. When I was a boy, my dad coached my Little League baseball team. Before each game, he would have us all sit on the bench and visualize hitting the baseball, running the bases, making great catches, and winning the game.

My dad often said that to be prepared to win the game, first, you must play through the entire game in your mind and see yourself winning. Then, you are prepared to play optimally on the field.

Those principles are not just limited to sports and performance on the field of play. Many professional athletes perform the visualization exercises while recovering from an injury in an effort to speed the healing process. While we are visualizing a certain activity, the brain does not recognize the difference between fantasy and reality. As a result, the same area of the brain that receives input during an actual event is also firing and receiving input during the visualization exercises. This is important, because as those centers of the brain fire, they cause the nerves to the muscles to fire, which speeds the healing process.

The mind-body connection is a growing area of interest in healthcare. After years of focusing completely on testing, prescription medication, and surgical procedures, the broader medical community is realizing that a patient's mindset has a direct correlation to the treatment outcome. Some of the early tests revealed the "healing power" of the mind. These were double blind studies performed where some of the test subjects were given real medications and some were given placebos. High numbers of the subjects given placebos had improved results. Their improvement was attributed to their belief in what they were given, and that it could heal them.

These studies coined the phrase "placebo effect." Obviously, there is something much more important going on in healing—it is the power of the mind. Treating the complete person is an effective adjunct to any treatment. Patient mind power is something I have used for years in treating all my patients, and I have seen that they respond more quickly and have better results.

Occasionally, I have a patient who is resistant to the idea of visualization. A few years ago, I treated a patient named Mary Ann. She was a middle-aged woman who had injured her back moving some large potted plants in her home. I did a complete examination, and as I asked questions about her medical history, I noticed that she was relating extremely negative aspects of her life and her health. She communicated that her life was awful and no one understood how she felt or sympathized with her condition. She also said that no one wanted to help her with anything. She blamed family, friends, other doctors, and anyone else she could think of for her problems.

Mary Ann was resistant to the idea of visualization. She could not imagine life without pain or struggle. She actively chose to view every person and event in her life as negative. Initially, I had limited improvement with Mary Ann, and she was pessimistic about the improvement she did experience.

Again, I sat down with her and discussed the importance of a positive attitude and the power of the visualization exercises. Mary Ann finally admitted to me that she was not following the recommendations and was not performing the exercise because she felt "stupid" doing them, and she did not continue the exercises. After explaining the importance of the exercises in both her health and her life, she finally agreed to begin again. From that point forward, her health improved as did her attitude toward life. These improvements were dramatic steps forward, and I am happy to report that her life changed in more than just physical improvement—this also helped improve her quality of life and the quality of her relationships. She had become a much happier and a more delightful person. It took a change in the way she viewed both her condition and her world to make a change, but the change was palpable.

As strange as it sounds, some of the patients I treat may have an emotional attachment to their pain. It is as if they do not want to let it go. The pain is one thing they have grown to count on and know as a constant. It becomes their purpose to discuss their condition with anyone who will listen. Everyone in the family becomes part of the suffering. This could be the natural part of the pain experience for some, but for others, health maladies may be an emotional crutch that excuses them from actively participating in life.

Other patients refuse to talk about their suffering with anyone. Perhaps, some feel there is no point in talking, as no one will understand anyway. Because pain is both a physical and psychological experience, there is a range of responses to pain. Patients who do not talk about their problems are the patients who need the visualization exercises the most, because if they cannot see it in their mind, they will certainly never achieve it in their lives.

## Supportive Studies

MORE STUDIES SUPPORTING the link between the mind and the body are presented every day. A study from the UCLA School of Medicine reported in the July 2008 issue of *Science Centric* that stress and negative emotions have a physical impact on the immune system. The protective end caps of cells, known as telomeres, remain long in those who have a positive outlook and less stress. Telomeres are indicators of the cell's ability to heal, and they show a direct link to our ability to stay well.

Another study, reported in the journal *Applied Psychophysiology and Biofeedback* in June 2001, used 20 subjects, all of whom had conditions that produced low white blood cell counts. These included patients with cancer, AIDS, and other autoimmune deficiencies. They used visualization and relaxation techniques each day, and after 90 days, all the subjects showed significant improvement in white blood cell counts. This shows a direct correlation between what we are thinking and our body's healing abilities.

# Expectation

WHEN I AM discussing treatment expectations with patients, I need to be certain we are talking about the same thing. The expectations of patients are an important part of their care, and I address this immediately. As an example, I explain to the patients who have had a back or neck problem for years that I am not going to be able to return their spine to that of a 20-year old, because there is a more significant degeneration now than when they were 20. It is important to know where the patient's mind is and what a starting perspective is. As the treatment progresses and pain diminishes, some patients forget how badly they felt before, and thus their expectations may rise to unrealistic levels.

I had such a conversation with a patient recently. She is in her mid-seventies, and I have treated her for many years. Her back pain has long since been resolved. Occasionally, I treat her for supportive care. She told me she was upset because she was limited in what she was able to do. After a long discussion about this "problem," I pointed out that her frustration was about attempting activities that people half her age have trouble doing.

One of my favorite stories of a patient who experienced the opposite life change is Ruby, a 63-year-old grandmother. Ruby had become very comfortable in her life. Her routine included gardening, having the grandkids over every Sunday, and meeting her friend for lunch on occasion. She did not socialize much or go anywhere outside her set routines. That particular winter, we had an extended ice storm, and Ruby had slipped on her porch and injured her lower back.

Ruby's injury made her almost housebound. When I first met with Ruby, she told me that she felt she had aged 20 years and was afraid her back injury would be permanent. I had Ruby start on positive visualizations immediately, and she quickly responded to treatment.

It was not long before she was traveling abroad and taking cruises. Her injury and her recovery had highlighted to her that her good health is to be treasured and enjoyed. She is bubbly and positive, and this attitude has the effect of making her seem much younger than her 63 years. Many times, life gives what we expect to get. The same can be applied when recovering from an injury or dealing with a degenerative disease.

I have another patient named Jarrod who had severe degeneration in the lumbar spine and was in his mid-fifties the first time I met with him. He brought an MRI for me to review. I have to admit that it made me do a double take. The degeneration I saw in his spine was severe, and he had bone spurring off the front and back of the vertebrae. Jarrod had a curve in his spine (scoliosis) that caused muscle spasm and chronic pain as well, and scoliotic curve may have been the cause of the degeneration. He was adamant that he did not want surgery. I agreed to do what I could, although this was such a serious condition there could have been limitations to the care. Jarrod had been a builder his entire life, and he refused to let his condition slow him down. He used this same determination and responded very well to treatment. During the course of his care, Jarrod began developing an entire housing development, and he amazed me with his positive attitude.

I see many patients with ongoing degeneration in their spines that is caused by osteoarthritis, and I see others with damage to nerves, such as diabetic neuropathy. It is important for patients to understand that they may have a problem that is entirely unrelated to their disc condition, or, they may have a degenerative hip-related condition that is causing some of their pain.

When I see patients with unrelated conditions, I discuss their treatment alternatives, and I note that they have complicating factors that will not respond to the DRS Protocol™. It is important for patients to understand they might have more than one condition that is playing a role in their symptoms. However, patients who have complicating factors can still achieve outstanding results for a disc-related condition with the DRS Protocol™.

The United States ranks number one in the use of surgery to treat back and neck pain. However, there are practitioners, including medical facilities, who offer treatment with spinal decompression. Not all facilities offer the complete DRS Protocol™ that I have developed. Many doctors simply treat with a spinal decompression table and offer a fixed number of treatments for a particular diagnosis. They are treating the diagnosis with a cookie-cutter approach, and they are not considering the overall patient. The DRS Protocol™ is customized for each patient and the specific condition. Each office is different and offers a different treatment program, and unless doctors have been trained by me, they do not offer the DRS Protocol™. As a side note: more and more doctors are being trained in the DRS Protocol™, so it is possible you may have a doctor in your area that has been trained. It is worth investigating.

## A Positive Experience for Patients

EXPECTATION IS VERY important to create a positive experience with your doctor, and my office offers the DRS Protocol™. The DRS Protocol™ is patient-centered healthcare and focuses on the complete patient, not just a symptom or area of disease. With this approach, I am able to determine and customize the best treatment options for each individual patient to ensure my office provides the gold standard of care and keeps its main focus on the patient. My goal is to have my patients' healthcare experiences be as positive, easy, and comfortable as possible.

I explain from the beginning that the patient will be an active participant in the care, and not just an observer. This can be a very different relationship from what some patients may have experienced in other healthcare offices. It is not uncommon for patients to be ignored or pushed out of their own healthcare decision-making process. Patients can become disillusioned by the lack of answers, attention, and compassion, as well as the great deal of time that must be invested in a doctor's waiting room. They may feel like a number.

The experience for the patient through the course of the DRS Protocol™ is a very comforting one. When treating for a low back problem, patients begin care by being placed on a spinal decompression table and lying on their back with a harness system around the pelvis, the thoracic spine, and rib cage. As a computerized distractive force is applied to the pelvic harnesses, the patient will feel a gentle pulling sensation in and about the lumbar spine. Treatment is directed to the patient's particular disc level of injury by adjusting the angle of force. The force is applied from a specific angle that is dependent upon the disc level being treated, and this varies from patient to patient. The amount of force to be applied is customized to each patient's individual condition and weight.

When treating the cervical spine, the amount of distractive force is again formulated based on the patient's condition and size, and will be significantly lower than the force for the lumbar spine. Cervical patients are also placed on a decompression table lying on their back. The patient's head and neck are stabilized in a cradle that extends around the back of the skull, or the occiput, and a very gentle distractive force is applied to the particular disc level, as noted above.

After finishing with the spinal decompression portion of care, the patient then undergoes separate physical therapy modalities, such as electrical stimulation, ultrasound, low level laser, ice/heat, and others (depending on what that particular patient's needs are), to reduce inflammation further while allowing the body to release its own natural painkillers, and allowing the body to heal.

Stabilization is the goal, and is not only the result of the disc healing, but also the result of exercise and nutrition used in conjunction with the rest of the treatment to help rebuild and strengthen the body.

During a short, beginning phase of care, patients are treated on a daily basis. Thereafter, the frequency decreases dependent upon their progress. My mindset, about treatment and everything I do in my office, is to look at each patient as an individual and base care on the individual situation.

There are many elements of the protocol. The DRS Protocol™ is not just a treatment using a particular type of spinal decompression table or therapies, it includes the positive experiences for a patient—from the first telephone call to my office to the complete course of the patient's care. All elements are involved in the success of the care.

Over time, I have treated many patients who were previously treated by another doctor with spinal decompression, without having achieved the best results. When patients receive treatment with the DRS Protocol™, they quickly realize that their care is much more involved. Their response to care is a positive outcome.

# CHAPTER 8

*A Life Without Pain*

# CHAPTER EIGHT

## *A Life Without Pain*

When someone is suffering from back or neck pain, there is no reason to be fearful of treatment and to continue living in pain. There is a successful and noninvasive alternative—the DRS Protocol™. My purpose in writing *Surgery not Included is to inform both patients and healthcare providers of the successful, nonsurgical option of the DRS Protocol™. This information is intended to inform those suffering from chronic pain that surgery is not their only option. Their treatment path does not need to be long, frustrating, and full of mediocre results.

One such case was Gavin. When I first examined Gavin, he was skeptical, angry, and having severe back pain. He had been to several doctors and two surgeons. Each one told him he absolutely had to have surgery. By the time he came to me, he was not sleeping due to his discomfort, and he was short-tempered and borderline abusive. He was what I would call "very difficult." Pain, anger, and fear can go hand-in-hand. When a chronic pain patient is told there is only one frightening solution—and it is not a good solution—frustration can boil over. Some take it out on everyone around them, including those who are trying to help.

It took a great deal of patience just to get through Gavin's evaluation. He even tested the patience of my staff, and they have been trained to work with patients who are in pain. It is sad to say how common this is, but I treat a high percentage of patients who have severe and chronic disc conditions, and they are suffering. Gavin had lived with pain for years. He had degenerative disc disease in his lower back, and he recently had fallen and exacerbated his back problem. He was experiencing shooting pain down both legs. I reviewed my exam and X-ray findings with him, and discussed treatment with the DRS Protocol™. Based on his experiences with doctors, he was more than reluctant. Nevertheless, he did not want surgery, so he said, "I'll try," all the while telling me he thought all "blanking" doctors were quacks. We talked about his attitude of implied failure. I told Gavin that "just trying" was not a strong enough commitment to produce the best outcome. He agreed, and we moved forward.

Within the first few treatments with the DRS Protocol™, the pain in both legs had significantly decreased, and Gavin was definitely getting around much better. After a few weeks, he seemed like a new man. He was finally sleeping, and being rested brightened his whole outlook. While it did not completely change his personality, it did improve his demeanor a great deal.

## *Loved Ones*

FAMILY MEMBERS OF patients can sometimes help and they can sometimes hurt. They can be so fed up with their loved one's complaints that they demand they come to see me. On the other hand, they can also be so convinced that surgery is the only way, that they discourage their loved ones from being assessed for the DRS Protocol™. In other cases, the family might discount altogether the patient's problem by inferring "it's all in your head." Or, for a number of reasons, they may actually interfere with the patient's decision-making.

Margie was such a patient. One of her dearest friends is also a patient of mine, and she strongly encouraged Margie to see me. It was winter, and she had a misstep off a curb, slipping on the ice. The result for Margie was a herniated disc accompanied by severe back and leg pain.

A close family member of Margie's was working for a surgeon and tried to convince her that treating with the DRS Protocol™ or with chiropractic care might cause severe damage or even stroke. Scientific studies clearly indicate that there is no significant risk for stroke from chiropractic care, and chiropractic treatment is safer than most medical treatments. DRS Protocol™ has no negative side effects. Sometimes other conditions, such as symptoms of what was assumed to be diabetic neuropathy, elevated blood pressure due to pain and stress, or incontinence, may clear up when the pressure on the nerves is removed.

Thankfully, Margie agreed to treatment, and within a few weeks, she made a full recovery with more than 95% improvement. Later, Margie's close family member became a patient of mine.

## The Simple Truth

I FOCUS ON providing a thorough layman's explanation to be absolutely certain my patients clearly understand the diagnosis and course of treatment. It is also important for patients to be able to explain their diagnosis and treatment to others. One of my first lessons in this as a young doctor occurred a number of years ago, when a woman named Ollie May came to see me. At the time, she was in her mid- to late-seventies and was a very sweet and delightful person. While examining her X-rays, I noticed that she had an abdominal aortic aneurysm. She had neglected to mention this in her medical history. Many times, patients do not understand why they need to tell a chiropractor about all health conditions and concerns. I asked her about the aneurysm, and she said she was aware of it and so was her cardiologist.

As I always do when patients have serious complicating conditions, I planned to contact Ollie May's cardiologist later that day, to discuss her treatment plan, confirming it would not interfere with any other treatment or problem with her aneurysm. When working with patients with an ongoing disease process such as heart disease, diabetes, aneurysm, transplant, and others, I look very closely at the treatment they are receiving for conditions outside of my care. When appropriate, I get clearance from their other physicians prior to beginning treatment. I send a complete report to the patient's specialists, so they are fully aware of the treatment I will be providing to a patient. This assures the patient that there is an adequate exchange of information about medical history, and that the treatment will be performed with the knowledge of everyone involved in care.

I knew I could help Ollie May with the pain she was experiencing in her back and legs. She left my office quite happy with this knowledge, but before my office could contact her cardiologist, I received a call from him. The conversation started with, "What exactly are you doing over there?"

Apparently, I had said something that Ollie May had interpreted somehow as my saying I could treat her aneurysm in addition to her disc. I had told her that I could treat her back condition despite the aneurysm. Ollie May had called her cardiologist and told him that I was going to treat her leg and back pain as well as fix her aneurysm, which was not the case. After a short explanation, the cardiologist approved treatment with the DRS Protocol™, and we had a good chuckle. However, I never forgot the lesson that if you do not explain things clearly and thoroughly, patients may fill in the blanks with the wrong information.

Never assume anything anyone repeats is 100% accurate—whether it is good or bad. Very often, patients come to my office for care after being seen by another doctor, and they tell me their back pain is the result of one leg being shorter than the other leg. In many cases, this is not the cause of the pain; it is a symptom of a biomechanical alteration. Each patient's experience, medical history, and current medical condition are unique, and there are no absolutes or across-the-board treatments when dealing with back and neck pain. Each situation must be evaluated by a qualified professional. Do not let someone else's opinion discourage you. Opinions and procedures may vary from city to city and region to region. There are alternatives available.

## *You Are in Charge*

MANY PATIENTS BELIEVE that they do not have control over their healthcare—but they do. It is true that insurance companies often dictate care. It is also true that patients are conditioned to go along with doctors' recommendations. Therefore, they just do not seek other treatment options. Some doctors are used to patients going along with recommendations without question. When a patient does ask questions, some doctors may become irritated because they are just not used to questions. A doctor should not forget that patients know their bodies and how they feel—doctors do not know everything about each specific patient, so just listening to a patient is critical.

I frequently treat patients with chronic pain who have been told by a doctor, at some point in their search for help, that perhaps stress or a relationship problem is the culprit, and perhaps there really is not a physical problem. This infers (if the doctor has not stated it outright) that "it is all in their head."

When the doctor, an authority figure, questions a person's reality, it can convince a patient that it is just destiny, and they have to live with pain and suffering. This is humiliating and stops some patients from investigating options because they are afraid they will experience the same embarrassing assumption again. Or they are told just to try a new medication and, "let's see what happens." This may be construed as a brush-off. It is discouraging, and again causes patients to question themselves.

How many times have you watched a commercial about a prescription drug, with a long, rapidly-read list of possible side effects, and have wondered who in their right mind would ever take that drug? The side effects are often worse than the condition the drugs are intended to cure. When a patient wants a doctor to provide a simple and fast solution, the doctor's decision is often affected by pharmaceutical-sponsored advertising.

Patients take some of the most harmful drugs because they believe they are needed, since a doctor prescribed them, and perhaps because their insurance covers it. Yet the entire list of the potential side effects may have never been fully explained, so some side effects come as a complete shock to the patient. I treat many patients who are taking so many medications that it is difficult to differentiate their true medical issues from drug side effects or drug interactions. A well known example is statins, which are prescribed for lowering cholesterol. Some doctors estimate that 15% of patients taking statins are affected in some manner. A prevalent symptom is mild-to-severe muscle cramping and spasms, and of a higher concern, are elevated liver enzymes. Frequently, I treat patients who have had to discontinue their cholesterol medications, and miraculously their leg pain goes away.

I will never forget a patient named Ellen who came in with a list of medications so long that I honestly had to wonder if her doctors truly had her best interests at heart. She was taking many medications, and some were prescribed just to combat the side effects of other medications. Ellen was taking stroke medications, blood thinners, diuretics, drugs to sleep, drugs to wake up, pain medications, drugs for heart disease and cholesterol, drugs for blood pressure, two for diabetes, one for neuropathy, one for diarrhea, and one for acid reflux.

This is not to say that Ellen did not have many health issues. But she never questioned the number or the types of medication that were prescribed. Every time she had a problem, she would go back to see a doctor or another specialist, and she would come back with another medication. In defense of her doctors, they were treating her conditions.

Doctors have to listen to their patients and pay attention to what they are being told. With the list of drugs Ellen was taking, one has to wonder if anyone was listening and how adding more drugs made sense. Even with the help of the Medicare or insurance prescription programs, there still have to be expenses involved in filling that many prescriptions, and there comes a point where it just does not make sense. The patient and the doctor must communicate.

My grandfather was told he had three months to live. He immediately stopped taking his medications since some had unpleasant side effects anyway. When my grandfather saw his doctor, he told the doctor that he had discontinued his medications. The doctor said that he needed to take, at least, the heart medications or he would die. My grandfather quickly replied, "You just told me I was going to die, and that stuff is expensive!" The interesting point is my grandfather felt better after discontinuing his medication. Yes, he finally did pass away, but nine months later. Obviously, patients should consult with their doctors before discontinuing any medications.

The lesson about Ellen is to ask questions. Even family members, who notice their loved ones are being prescribed more and more medications, should be proactive and ask some questions. The truth is that the body has tremendous abilities to heal without the long-term use of drugs. The problem with many prescription drugs is that they stop vital reactions and processes in the body. When that happens, there cannot be normal health, and there have to be side effects. Often these medications can interfere with the body's natural processes. Certain medications and even drug interactions can slow the healing process.

Taking charge of your healthcare and committing to gain knowledge about your body and how to heal naturally will decrease the need for prescriptions and invasive procedures for disc-related conditions. My main goal in writing *Surgery not Included is to provide the knowledge that many patients need to make informed healthcare decisions. Patients frequently come to my office and tell me what treatments their previous doctors have recommended. However, they rarely can tell me what their diagnosis was or what it meant. It is important to know exactly what is to be treated, and why, before agreeing to a procedure. Many times, the problem is simply with communication. Doctors do not always communicate effectively, if at all. Remember that the medical system does not allow much time for listening and eliciting information from patients, and patients do not always report properly and are afraid to ask questions. This alone can lead to unnecessary suffering. I take time to educate my patients so they know exactly what is wrong, that way, they can take an active role in their own care. Every person is unique and needs to be treated as such. Just because some doctors treat patients like numbers does not mean we should accept it.

The body is a wonderfully created machine and, if allowed, most disc conditions can heal more perfectly, given the proper environment, than anything done with invasive treatment can achieve. This is the philosophy of chiropractic care and the DRS Protocol™ for spinal decompression, and I teach this protocol to doctors across the country. We can help without inflicting trauma.

My goal is to get the patient well. I have dedicated my life to helping sick and suffering people. Through the years, I have had many employees who were registered nurses. Some had extensive experience in different healthcare settings, from the hospital ER to the family doctor. Each one has said the same thing: "I love working here; the office is full of happy people and they get well!"

## *Your Choices Matter*

MORE THAN 90% of overall health is due to lifestyle and environmental factors that influence our health. This means that most adults have an extraordinary amount of control over their own health through the choices made every day. This includes everything from avoiding those items that we know are detrimental, as well as following a balanced diet, and getting some form of exercise. There is much misinformation about what the body needs, what constitutes a healthy lifestyle, and what qualifies as a balanced diet. Double-check your sources.

In general terms, you cannot go wrong when buying organic meats, fruits, and vegetables, and staying away from processed foods. This is because nonorganic foods are treated with substances that are harmful to the body or that mimic hormones within the body, which can cause disease. The higher the quality of food you put into your body, the better you will feel and the fewer problems you will have. On occasion, when I mention this, I get the standard response from patients that organic is expensive and just too much trouble. Yet, when the cost of organic foods is compared to the cost of prescription drugs and medical procedures to treat the disease processes caused by pesticides, hormones, and other negative, external influences—then organic foods could be considered a bargain.

Smoking is detrimental to healing. Some studies indicate that there are over 2,000 chemicals in cigarette smoke, and these all cause problems with the way your body functions. Not only does it shorten your life span, it also severely inhibits your ability to recover from an injury. Smokers rarely achieve the best treatment outcomes. That is sad and unnecessary, which is why I discourage my patients' smoking. Even if I am able to discourage my patients from smoking for the duration of their treatment, they will have a greater advantage to achieve maximum healing.

The discontinuation of destructive habits, such as smoking or drinking alcohol excessively, coupled with encouraging positive aspects, such as exercise and eating an organic diet, can have tremendously positive long-term effects. One of the best actions anyone can take to improve health is to stop destructive or harmful habits. Working with our natural processes and paying attention when our body tells us something is wrong is also one of the best preventive strategies.

A frequent situation I encounter is patients who have allowed their pain condition to go on for years, and therefore, they have caused unnecessary damage. By listening to your body and getting help early, rather than waiting, you can have positive results.

One of my patients, named Jerry, worked as a truck driver for over 20 years. He was overweight, and the stress and strain of his job had resulted in on-and-off lower back pain. He had been suffering from back problems for more than 10 years. He popped ibuprofen as if it was candy, and he frequently slept sitting in a recliner, because his legs became numb when he lay down. Jerry did not feel the need to see a doctor about these problems, until he reached a point that his pain was interfering with his ability to work. This is very common, especially with men, and particularly if their pain has not been debilitating. They adjust to higher levels of pain, and if it does not keep them from working, they do not think it is bad enough to visit the doctor.

Jerry was just this type of guy. I see this often with farmers, construction workers, and truck drivers. All of them, and there are certainly others, are hard working, do not offer excuses, and have a strong work ethic. Yet, this is bad because the body is saying, "something is wrong." The body is trying to protect the spinal structure. This means increased swelling, more nerve damage, and more deterioration. Some of these changes will be permanent if not corrected in a timely fashion.

Jerry was treated with the DRS Protocol™ and had an excellent outcome with more than 90% improvement. He now recognizes that correcting his small back problems early will prevent debilitating ones later. It is this realization that causes many patients to refer their family members and friends for care. They understand that more severe problems are created by waiting.

## Focus on the "After"

WE HAVE ALL seen the advertising of the before-and-after photos of people who have had tremendous weight loss. I often wish I had something similar to show the dramatic changes we create in people's lives by helping their pain. Even though they appear the same on the outside, their attitudes and outlooks on life have changed. For those who are currently in pain and wondering if the DRS Protocol™ with spinal decompression may offer the answer, I would encourage them to focus on the "after." Much like the visualization exercises I give patients to perform, believing that he or she can get well and believing that there is a nonsurgical solution is the first step to living a full and pain-free life.

I often find that patients in pain resign themselves to their lives. They do not look ahead or think about tomorrow. Because they are in pain, they can focus only on today and getting through it. Before long, their lives turn inward and become like a daily grind of pain upon more pain. Usually after a few days of treatment with the DRS Protocol™, they begin to see beyond today, and then look forward to tomorrow. Before long, they are reviving lost dreams.

As I teach this protocol to other doctors, patients have more and more access to effective and safe alternatives that can give them back the lives they once had. I always ask my patients to rate their percentage of improvement. This is a way to compare their pain reduction, as opposed to their pain level when they started care. This allows them to realize the vast amount of progress they have made in a very short time. While I always emphasize that if you are 50 years old, you will not return to way you were physically when you were 20, you also will not feel as if you are 75 or 80. The goal is to get the patient to feel as well as possible for the given age and state of health, and in that respect, I have tremendous success.

## *You Partner in Healthcare*

WITHIN THE PAGES of this book, I have conveyed not only my medical knowledge and expertise, but also my philosophy in patient care. I feel very strongly that I am a partner with my patients on their journey to recovery. I am not a commander but a coach, an expert with the tools to help them to complete the process of becoming free from pain.

An important aspect of the DRS Protocol™ is that the patient is treated as a special human being. We all have wants, needs, and desires, and we consist of more than our physical bodies. When doctors ignore the emotional and spiritual aspects of what it is to be human, they shortchange the patient's overall health and just treat a symptom.

I believe the foundation of patient care is in the relationship between the doctor and patient, one that we build together. I have a strong commitment to seeing my patients through their care and to a positive outcome. I want to assure anyone who is suffering from back or neck pain that there is hope. You do not have to live in pain. Do not wait one more day to begin your new life, living free of pain and full of promise of a bright and active future. *Surgery not Included.

# GLOSSARY

**Acute pain:** Resulting from a specific incident of tissue damage as in, burning a finger on a hot iron.

**Alkaline phosphatase:** An enzyme originating from the liver, bone, or the placenta. This is released into the blood when an injury occurs and during bone growth.

**Allopathic doctors:** Medical doctors who use methods of treating disease by the use of agents that produce effects different from those the disease treated.

**Amputee:** Individual who has lost one or both legs due to trauma or disease.

**Amitriptyline:** A medication used to treat various forms of depression, pain associated with the nerves (neuropathic pain), and to prevent migraine headaches. It is sold in the United States under the brand names Elavil® and Endep® and also helps patients sleep.

**Anatomy:** The study of form. Gross anatomy involves structures that can be seen with the naked eye as opposed to microscopic anatomy (or histology) which involves structures seen under the microscope. Traditionally, both gross and microscopic anatomy have been studied in the first year of medical school in the U.S. The most celebrated textbook of anatomy in the English-speaking world is Gray's Anatomy, still a useful reference book.

**Aneurysm:** An area of an artery, vein, or the heart that has weakened and is bulging or threatening to rupture.

**Ankylosing spondylitis:** A type of arthritis that causes chronic inflammation of the spine and the sacroiliac joints. This can lead to pain and stiffness in the spinal region. This condition can lead to a natural fusion of the vertebrae causing total loss of motion in the spinal region.

**Arachnoiditis:** A debilitating condition characterized by severe stinging, burning pain, and neurologic problems.

**Arthritis:** Inflammation of a joint. There are well over 100 types of arthritis, which can leave the joints inflamed resulting in stiffness, swelling, and pain.

**Articular cartilage:** Cartilage that covers the articular surfaces of bones.

**Aspirin:** The common name for acetylsalicylic acid. Patients often use this as their first line of pain relief.

**Atherosclerosis:** Progressive thickening and hardening of the walls of arteries as a result of fat deposits.

**Bacteria:** Single-celled microorganisms, which can exist either as independent organisms or as parasites. Bacterial infections can range from mild to life threatening. Infection is a common surgical complication.

**Biological barrier:** A biological barrier forms when the cut that forms the scar tissue is made with a sharp object (such as a scalpel) leaving an impenetrable wall that will not heal properly over time. To understand this further, we can compare it to transplanting a plant to a large pot. If you try to replant the plant in a larger pot without first roughening up the root ends (from a clean cut), the roots will not take because in essence they have created a biological barrier.

**Blood:** Fluid in the body that transports all the elements necessary for life including water, nutrient, minerals and oxygen. The discs between the vertebrae absorb these essential items through a process called diffusion.

**Blood pressure:** The pressure placed on the arterial wall by the blood as it circulates through the body. Elevated blood pressure is an indicator of possible heart disease or risk of stroke.

**Bone:** Bone is the hard substance that forms the skeleton of the human body. Its composition is mainly calcium phosphate and calcium carbonate. Bone also serves as a storage area for calcium, playing a large role in calcium balance in the blood.

**Bowel:** Another name for the intestine. The small bowel and the large bowel are the small intestine and large intestine and process all the food we take in. Some pain medications can cause gastrointestinal bleeds.

**Brain:** The part of the central nervous system that is located within the skull. The brain functions as the primary receiver, organizer and distributor of information for the body. Pain is received and processed in the brain and each person perceives pain differently.

**Calcitonin:** A hormone produced by the thyroid gland that lowers the levels of calcium and phosphate in the blood. This hormone promotes the formation of new bone.

**Cannula:** A tube inserted into a bodily cavity that may be used to administer a substance.

**Cartilage:** Tissue with a firm, rubbery consistency that cushions bones at joints. Tendons and ligaments are made of a more flexible type of cartilage and connect muscles with bones and make up other parts of the body, such as the larynx and the exterior of the ears.

**CAM (Complementary and Alternative Medicine):** Complementary and alternative medicine is a group of diverse medical and healthcare systems, practices, and products that are not generally considered part of conventional medicine.

**CAT scan:** The CAT (Computerized Axial Tomography) scan, also known as the CT (computed tomography) scan, is an X-ray technique that produces pictures representing a detailed cross section of body's tissue.

**Chronic pain:** Pain that has lasted beyond the 3-6 month time frame for tissue healing. This type of pain is ongoing and more constant than acute pain.

**Complication:** This is an additional problem that arises following a procedure, surgery or treatment. This can add to the difficulty of recovery for the patient or extend the recovery period.

**Compression fracture:** A hairline break in a bone cause by hitting another bone and being "compressed."

**Cortisone:** This is an adrenocorticoid hormone, a naturally occurring hormone made by and secreted by the adrenal cortex, the outer part of the adrenal gland. Cortisone is useful in reducing inflammation.

**Cauda equina:** A bundle of spinal nerve roots that arise from the bottom end of the spinal cord.

**Cox 2 inhibitors:** Drugs used to treat the pain and swelling of arthritis inflammation.

**Dexa scan:** Bone density scan that gives an actual risk score.

**Degenerative arthritis:** This is also known as osteoarthritis, this type of arthritis is caused by inflammation of cartilage in the joints and an eventual breakdown and loss of that cartilage. This is the most common type of arthritis.

**Diabetes:** A chronic disease characterized by high glucose levels within the body. Can cause diabetic neuropathy as the glucose levels make the nerves deteriorate.

**Diagnosis:** The identification of a particular disease or condition.

**Disc:** In relation to the spine, this is an intervertebral disc, a disc-shaped piece of specialized tissue that separates the bones of the spine and prevents them rubbing against one another.

**Discogram:** A diagnostic test where the doctor injects dye into the disc. A very painful test that also destroys the disc.

**Discectomy:** Excision, in part or whole, of an intervertebral disc.

**Dysesthesia:** Impairment of sensitivity especially to touch.

**Epidural space:** The outermost part of the spinal canal.

**Epidural injection:** Medication delivered into the spinal cavity. For back pain, usually a mixture of anti-inflammatory and pain medication.

**EMG (Electromyography):** Involves testing the electrical activity of muscles. It is a test used to evaluate electrical impulses from the nerves.

**ED (Erectile dysfunction):** Is the inability of a man to maintain a firm erection long enough to have sex.

**Estrogen:** Estrogen is a female hormone produced by the ovaries. Phytoestrogens can cause undesirable effects and are found in soy products. Estrogen deficiency can lead to osteoporosis.

**Extremity:** These are used to refer to the hands and feet. Many patients have tingling or numbness in their extremities.

**Examination:** The doctor/patient time used for evaluating a person's physical condition and medical history.

**Facet joints:** Facet joints occur in pairs at the back of each vertebra. The facet joints link the vertebrae directly above and below to form a working unit that permits movement of the spine.

**Foramina:** A small opening in the bone through which nerves pass

**Fracture:** A break in bone or cartilage. Degenerative diseases and loss of calcium can make bones prone to fracture.

**Functional scoliosis:** A structurally normal spine that appears to have a lateral curve (scoliosis).

**Herniated disc:** Rupturing of the intervertebral disc tissue that separates the vertebral bones of the spinal column. The tissue herniates out of position and can press on the nerves of the spine.

**Herniation:** Abnormal extrusion of tissue through an opening. For example, an intervertebral disc located between vertebrae can push out of position and press against nerves.

**Hormone:** A chemical substance produced in the body that controls and regulates the activity of certain cells or organs.

**Iliac:** Pertaining to the ilium, the lowest part of the abdominal regions.

**Incontinence:** Urinary incontinence refers to the inability to keep urine in the bladder. Nerve compression sometimes causes incontinence problems.

**Inflammation:** An immune response to injury, irritation or infection. Inflammation causes swelling, redness and pain.

**Injury:** Trauma inflicted on the body inducing acute pain or damage to tissues.

**Joint:** The point where two bones come together and allow articulation of the body. Joints contain fibrous connective tissue and cartilage.

**Laminectomy:** A surgical procedure in which the posterior arch of a vertebra is removed. Laminectomy is done to relieve pressure on the spinal cord or on the nerve roots that emerge from the spinal canal. The procedure may be used to treat a slipped or herniated disc or to treat spinal stenosis.

**Ligament:** A sheet or band of tough, fibrous tissue connecting bones or cartilages at a joint or supporting an organ.

**Low back pain:** Pain in the region know as the lower back can indicate problems with the lumbar spine, the discs between the vertebrae, the ligaments around the spine and discs, the spinal cord and nerves, muscles of the lower back, internal organs of the pelvis and abdomen, or the skin covering the lumbar area.

**Lumbar radiculopathy:** Nerve irritation caused by damage to the discs between the vertebrae. Damage to the disc occurs because of normal wear and tear of the outer ring of the disc, injury, or both. As a result, the gel like center portion of the disc can herniated through the outer ring of the disc and press against the spinal cord or its nerves as they exit the bony spinal column. This can cause the commonly recognized pain known as sciatica that shoots down the leg.

**Lumbar strain:** A stretching injury to the ligaments, tendons, and/or muscles of the low back. The stretching incident results in microscopic tears of varying degrees in these tissues. Lumbar strain is one of the most common causes of low back pain. The injury can occur because of overuse, improper use, or trauma. It is classified as "acute" if it has been present for days to weeks. If the strain lasts longer than 3 months, it is referred to as "chronic."

**Lumbar vertebrae:** There are five lumbar vertebrae. These vertebrae are situated between the thoracic vertebrae and the sacral vertebrae in the spinal column. The five lumbar vertebrae are represented by the symbols L1 through L5.

**Lymph fluid:** An almost colorless fluid that travels through vessels called lymphatics in the lymphatic system and carries cells that help fight infection and disease.

**MRI:** Acronym for magnetic resonance imaging, which produces images of the soft tissues of the body by detecting differences in tissue density.

**MRSA bacteria:** Drug resistant strain of flesh eating bacteria known to thrive in many hospitals. This infection can be a complication of surgery.

**Muscle:** Muscle is the tissue of the body, which primarily creates movement. There are three types of muscle in the body. Muscle that is responsible for moving extremities and external areas of the body is called skeletal muscle. Heart muscle is called cardiac muscle. Muscle that is in the walls of arteries and bowel is called smooth muscle.

**Muscle-guarding:** Spasm of the muscles that occurs after a back or neck injury. A protection mechanism of the body.

**Musculoskeletal:** Relating to or involving the muscles and the skeleton.

**Myelogram:** An X-ray of the spinal cord after a contrast dye is injected.

**Myelofibrosis:** Fibrosis (spontaneous scarring) of the bone marrow.

**NSAIDs (nonsteroidal anti-inflammatory drugs):** These include aspirin, ibuprofen (Advil® and Motrin®), naproxen sodium (Aleve®), and ketoprofen (Orudis KT®).

**Nerve:** Fibers made up of trillions of individual nerve cells that transmit electrical impulses from the body to the brain for interpretation.

**Nerve ablation:** Destruction of the nerve through radio waves.

**Nerve conduction velocity (NCV):** Tests the electrical function of the nerve itself.

**Nerve root:** Nerve branching off from the spinal cord.

**Neurological:** Medical specialty concerned with treating the nervous system: Brain, spinal cord, and nerves.

**Neuropathy:** Pain along the path of a nerve.

**Off label drug use:** The practice of prescribing pharmaceuticals for a purpose outside the scope of a drug's approved label.

**Osteoarthritis:** A type of arthritis caused by inflammation, breakdown, and eventual loss of cartilage in the joints.

**Osteomyelitis:** Inflammation of the bone due to infection. Osteomyelitis can be a complication of surgery or injury, although infection can also reach bone tissue through the bloodstream. Both the bone and the bone marrow may be infected. Symptoms include deep pain and muscle spasms in the area of inflammation, and fever.

**Osteoporosis:** Reduction in bone mass due to depletion of calcium and bone protein. Osteoporosis can make the bones fragile and prone to fractures, which are often slow to heal and heal poorly. It is more common in older adults, particularly post-menopausal women; in patients on steroids; and in those who take steroidal drugs. Unchecked osteoporosis can lead to changes in posture, physical abnormality and decreased mobility.

**Orthopedic:** Specialty involved in taking care of the skeletal system.

**Pain:** An unpleasant feeling that can range from mild, localized discomfort to agony. Pain has both physical and emotional components. The physical part of pain results from nerve stimulation. Pain is carried to the brain along nerve fibers for interpretation. Every person perceives pain differently.

**Paraspinal Muscles:** Muscles adjacent to the spine that support the movement of the spine.

**Pelvis:** The lower part of the abdomen located between the hip bones.

**Percutaneous:** Under the skin.

**Phantom pain:** The sensation that the injury is still present long after the site has healed. In amputees, the sensation that the limb is still there long after amputation.

**Physical therapy:** Rehabilitative healthcare that uses specially designed exercises and equipment to help patients regain or improve their physical abilities. Physical therapy is one of the first treatments given to back pain sufferers.

**Prostaglandins:** One of a number of hormone-like substances that participate in a wide range of body functions.

**Protein:** A large molecule composed of one or more chains of amino acids in a specific order determined by the base sequence of nucleotides in the DNA coding for the protein.

**Radiate:** To start in one location and spread out. Pain may radiate from one point and affect several parts of the body.

**Radiculopathy:** Any disease of the spinal nerve roots and spinal nerves.

**Rotation and flexion and extension:** This refers to a range of motion.

**Sacrum:** Made up of fused sacral vertebrae, the sacrum is the large heavy bone located at the base of the spine. The sacrum is located in the spinal column, between the lumbar vertebrae and the coccyx. It is somewhat triangular in shape and is largely the back wall of the pelvis. The female sacrum is wider and less curved than the male to allow for childbirth.

**Scar tissue:** The fibrous tissue that the body creates to replace damaged skin is called a scar. Scars are also know as cicatrices and are formed as a biological response for repairing skin and other tissue damage in the human body

**Sciatica:** Pain resulting from inflammation of or pressure on, the sciatic nerve. This type of pain is typically felt from the lower back to under the buttocks, radiating down below the knee. Sciatica frequently results from a herniated disc directly pressing on the nerve, but can be cause by any irritation or inflammation.

**Scoliosis:** Lateral curvature of the spine.

**Somatovisceral referred pain:** The combination of nerve pain from organs, skin and musculoskeletal origins.

**Spasm:** Involuntary repeated awkward jerking movements. A muscle spasm cause tremendous pain as the muscles contract. Nerve pain in the spine can cause the surrounding muscles to spasm.

**Spinal cord:** The main bundle of nerve tissue that is connected to the brain and lies within the vertebral canal. Thirty-one pairs of spinal nerves originate in the spinal cord: 8 cervical, 12 thoracic, 5 lumbar, 5 sacral, and 1 coccygeal. The spinal cord and the brain make up the central nervous system. The spinal cord consists of nerve fibers that transmit impulses to and from the brain.

**Spinal fluid:** Fluid located within the spinal column that cushions and protects the spine.

**Spinal nerve:** One of the nerves that originates in the spinal cord.

**Spinal stenosis:** Narrowing of the open spaces in the spine. This can cause compression of the nerve roots or spinal cord by bony spurs or soft tissues, such as discs, in the spinal canal. This occurs most often in the lumbar spine (in the low back) but also occurs in the cervical spine (in the neck) and less often in the thoracic spine (in the upper back).

**Spinal tumor:** A tumor located within the spinal column that compresses the nerves of the spine.

**Spine:** The column of bone known as the vertebral column, which runs down the middle of the back and surrounds and protects the spinal cord. The spine can be categorized according to level of the body: cervical spine (neck), thoracic spine (upper and middle back), and lumbar spine (lower back).

**Spinous process:** A slender projection from the back of a vertebra, which is where muscles and ligaments are attached.

**Spondylitis:** Inflammation of one or more of the vertebrae of the spine. Diffuse inflammation of the spine is seen in the disease ankylosing spondylitis. Localized spondylitis is seen with infections of a certain area of the spine, such as in Pott's disease.

**Spondylosis:** Degeneration of the disc spaces between the vertebrae. This finding in the spine is commonly associated with osteoarthritis.

**Subluxation:** When one or more bones of the spine move out of position and cause pressure on the nerves.

**Surgery:** Surgery is the work done by a surgeon. An operation to correct a problem.

**Tendon:** The tissue that attaches muscle to bone. A tendon is flexible, but also fibrous and tough. When a tendon becomes inflamed, the condition is referred to as tendinitis or tendonitis. Inflamed tendons are at risk for rupture.

**TENS:** Transcutaneous Electric Neural Stimulator unit, which helps interrupt pain messages to the brain. Developed by C. Norman Shealy, M.D., Ph.D.

**Tethers:** Imagine that when performing surgery you need to cut through tissue to get to the area you want to affect. This tissue is not just connected in the area that is cut, but can travel throughout the body. When the tissue is sutured or stitched up, this can create a tethering effect that can in essence cause painful symptoms throughout the body.

**Tissue meninges:** The system of membranes that envelops the central nervous system. The meninges consist of three layers: the dura mater, the arachnoid mater, and the pia mater. The primary function of the meninges and of the cerebrospinal fluid is to protect the central nervous system.

**Trauma:** Any injury, whether physically or emotionally inflicted. Trauma is a serious or critical bodily injury, wound, or shock. This definition is often associated with trauma medicine practiced in emergency rooms.

**Vertebra:** A vertebra is one of 33 bony segments that form the spinal column of humans. There are 7 cervical, 12 thoracic, 5 lumbar, 5 sacral (fused into 1 sacrum bone) and 4 coccygeal (fused into 1 coccyx bone).

**Vertebrae:** The preferred plural of vertebra.

**Vessel:** A tube in the body that carries fluids: blood vessels or lymph vessels.

**X-ray:** High-energy radiation with waves shorter than those of visible light. In low doses, X-rays are used for making images that help to diagnose disease, and in high doses to treat cancer.

# ANNOTATED BIBLIOGRAPHY

## Synopsis of Research on Cervical and Lumbar Decompression/Traction

Onel D et al. CT investigation of the effects of traction on lumbar herniation. Spine. 1989;14:82-90. Thirty patients with lumbar herniations underwent traction in a CT scanner at >50% body weight for 20 minutes. Herniation retraction occurred in 70% and good clinical improvements were seen in over 93%. The authors concluded improved blood flow was the source of healing and that the traction did not create negative intradiscal pressure due to inadequate traction force.

Tilaro F. Canadian Journal of Clinical Medicine. 1998;5:1-7. Decompression therapy significantly reduced intradiscal pressure. Promoting retraction of the herniation, improving diffusion gradient into the disc that allows nutrients and healing.

Note: controversy whether decompression actually occurs and if it occurs how functional is it once the patient stands or sits and weight bearing reoccurs.

Nachemson A. Intradiscal pressure. Journal of Neurosurgery 1995;82:1095. Criticized Tilaro experimental setup saying that there wasn't a control group, patients were not randomly assigned, and lacked follow-up scores. Reported the study was not clinically meaningful due to these flaws.

Saal JA, Saal JS. Nonoperative treatment of herniated lumbar disc with radiculopathy (leg pain). Spine. 1989;14(4):431-437. Fifty-eight subjects; 86% had good-to-excellent results with inclusive conservative program to include traction and trunk stabilization exercises.

Mathews JA et al. Manipulation and traction for lumbago and sciatica. Physio Pract. 1988;4:201. Eight-five percent reported substantial relief with a controlled trial of traction combined with manipulative therapy. Traction force applied at 100 pounds for 20 minutes.

Constatoyannis C et al. Intermittent cervical traction for radiculopathy due to large volume herniations. Journal of Manipulative and Physiological Therapeutics. 2002;25(3). Four subjects displayed complete resolution of symptoms after three weeks of cervical traction.

Erhard R et al. Intermittent cervical traction and thoracic manipulation for management of mild cervical compressive myelopathy attributed to cervical herniated disc: A case series. Journal of Orthopaedic and Sports Physical Therapy. 2004;34(11). Intermittent cervical traction and manipulation of the thoracic spine was useful for the reduction of pain scores and level of disability in patients with mild cervical compressive myelopathy attributed to herniated disc.

Shealy N, Leroy P. New concepts in back pain management. AJPM. 1998;(1)20:239-241. The application of supine lumbar traction altering the angle of pull from 10° to 30° and progression to peak force enhanced distraction at specific levels in the lumbar spine. Increase distraction at L5/S1 with 10° angle of pull and L3 with 30° angle of pull.

Weatherall VF. Comparison of electrical activity in the sacrospinalis musculature during traction in two different positions. Journal of Orthopaedic and Sports Physical Therapy. 1995;(8):382-390. EMG electrical activity shown to be similar in the prone versus supine positions.

Letchuman R, Deusinger RH. Comparison of sacrospinalis myoelectric activity and pain levels in patients undergoing static and intermittent lumbar traction. Spine. 1993;18(10):1361-1365. Improved comfort and less muscle guarding noted in the intermittent traction group.

Nanno M. Effects of intermittent cervical traction on muscle pain. EMG and flowmetric studies on cervical paraspinals. Journal of Nippon Medical School. April 1994;61(2):137-47. Intermittent cervical traction was shown to be effective in relieving pain, improving blood flow and increasing myoelectric signals in the effected muscles.

Chung TS, Lee YJ et al. Reducibility of cervical herniation: Evaluation at MRI during cervical traction with a nonmagnetic device. Radiology. December 2002;225(3):895-900. Twenty-nine patients and seven healthy volunteers had intermittent cervical traction while in MR. Substantial increase in vertebral length was seen. Full herniation reduction in three patients and partial reduction in eighteen was reported.

Hseuh TC et al. Evaluation of the effects of pulling angle and force on intermittent cervical traction. Journal of the Formosan Medical Association. 1991;90(12):1234-1249. Traction under 30° created longest gap at C4-6 and under 35° created longest gap at C6-T1.

Gionis TA, Groteke E. Spinal decompression. Clinical study evaluating the effect of nonsurgical intervention on symptoms of spine patients with herniated and degenerative disc disease. Orthopedic Technology Review. November to December 2003;5(6):36. Of 219 subjects, 86% reported completed resolution of symptoms and 84% of this group remained pain-free for three months.

# ENDNOTES

1.  Ramos G, Martin W. Effects of vertebral axial decompression on intradiscal pressure. Journal of Neurosurgery. September 1994;81:350-353.

2.  Onel D et al. CT investigation of the effects of traction on lumbar herniation. Spine. 1989;14:82-90.

3.  Nachemson A. Intradiscal pressure. Journal of Neurosurgery. 1995;82:1095.

4.  Tilaro F, Miskovich D. The effects of vertebral axial decompression on sensory nerve dysfunction in patients with low back pain and radiculopathy. Canadian Journal of Clinical Medicine. 1999;6(1):1-8.

5.  Ramos G, Martin W. Effects of vertebral axial decompression on intradiscal pressure. Journal of Neurosurgery. September 1994;81:350-353.

6.  Mathews JA et al. Manipulation and traction for lumbago and sciatica. Physio Pract. 1988;4:201.

7.  Chen YG, Li FB, Huang CD. Biomechanics of traction for lumbar disc prolapse. Chinese Ortho. January 1994;(1):40-2.

# RECOMMENDED RESOURCES

## Dr. Rick Busch Will Tell You...

# "FORMULA 303 BREAKS THE CHAIN OF PAIN AND NERVOUS TENSION NINE PROVEN WAYS"

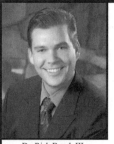

Dr. Rick Busch III

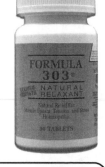

**#1  RELAXES...** Muscle Spasms
**#2  RELIEVES...** Tension and Stress
**#3  EASES...** Lower Back Pain
**#4  SOOTHES...** PMS and Menstrual Cramps
**#5  LOOSENS...** Tight Muscles
**#6  CALMS...** Nervousness
**#7  REDUCES...** Leg Cramps
**#8  QUIETS...** Pulled Muscles
**#9  COMFORTS...** Neck and Shoulder Pain

**Over 6,000 Chiropractors have recommended And used FORMULA 303... Here's a few things They have said about this proven formula...**

*"FORMULA 303 is the only product I have used over the past ten years...I feel there is no better product and my patients love it".*

*"FORMULA 303 works better that any similar product I have used in my 28 years of practice."*

*"FORMULA 303 works better than anything else I've used for muscle spasms, tension, and stress."*

*" I feel everyone can benefit from FORMULA 303... Especially here in New York City where 'stress' is our middle name."*

*WHAT MAKES THIS MAXIMUM STRENGTH HOMEOPATHIC FORMULA THE FIRST CHOICE OF CHIROPRACTORS !!*

**VALERIAN ROOT** 6 parts (quad strength) 1X-valerian works naturally to relieve muscle spasms and nervousness with a resulting calming effect on the system.

**PASSIFLORA** 3 parts (quad strength) 1X-passiflora contains unique natural flavonoids that are believed to be responsible in helping to relax the effects of anxiety while helping to relieve muscle tension throughout the body.

**MAGNESIUM CARBONATE** one part 1X-magnesium is an essential mineral for muscle relaxation, fighting PMS, restless legs and muscle spasms.

**It is 100% safe WITHOUT** interfering with your patient's natural functions or body chemistry.

Mfg. in our FDA Registered Facility using Good Manufacturing Practices (GMPs). Meets USP <2040> for disintegration for maximum bioavailability.

This "GUARANTEED POTENCY" symbol is your assurance of dependable, consistent quality and potency in every tablet

---

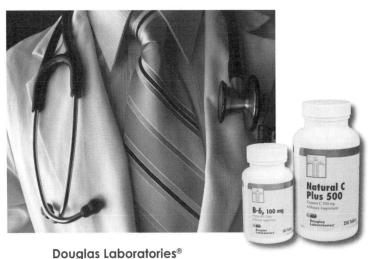

## Douglas Laboratories®

**Quality Nutritional Supplements Exclusively for Health Professionals**

### Raising the Standard
### With innovative, clinically backed formulas.

Our standards stand for quality of life: we provide the highest quality nutritional supplements available with the highest level of personal service—anywhere. For more than 50 years, Douglas Laboratories has provided a custom approach to nutrition and wellness that your patients won't find anywhere else. We continue to lead the industry with the largest and most innovative line of nutritional supplements, supported by science and clinical trials. Visit our website for our new in-office patients' education posters, easy online ordering and other innovative ideas designed to help your practice grow...douglaslabs.com.

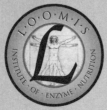
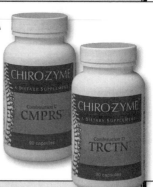

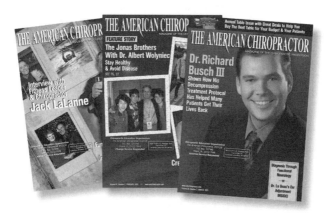

# THE AMERICAN CHIROPRACTOR
### MAGAZINE OF THE CHIROPRACTIC PROFESSION

## Committed to the Continuing Education and Advancement of the Chiropractic Professional

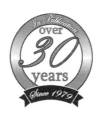

# *Surgery not Included
## FREEDOM
### from Chronic Neck and Back Pain

## Dr. Richard E. Busch III
5005 Riviera Court,
Fort Wayne, IN 46825

*Book Order Form*

**PERSONAL INFORMATION**

Name

Address

City                                      Suite / Apt #

Prov / State    Country                   Postal / Zip Code

Telephone Number                          Fax Number

Email

---

### Order Your Copy of the Book Today!

for only **$29.95**

---

**SHIPPING**

**Postage is calculated as follows:**
For the first book:
**US:** $6.50    ($3.00 for each
**CA:** $7.00    additional book)

**Please send payment and order to:**

**Dr. Richard E. Busch III**
5005 Riviera Court,
Fort Wayne, IN 46825

Ship To: (if different from above) —————————————————————————————

Credit Card Number: _____ Expiration Date: _____/_____/_____

Signature: _____ Visa; MC; AMEX; DSC (Circle one)

We accept: Check, Money Order,

---

*Thank you for your order.* | (888) 471-4090 | *DrBusch@SurgeryNotIncluded.com*

# ABOUT THE AUTHOR

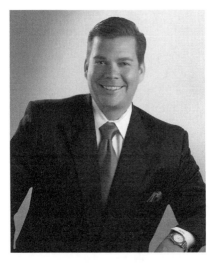

Dr. Richard E. Busch III, is the founder of the Busch Chiropractic Pain Center and cofounder of Freedom Awaits™. He is a nationally recognized chiropractor, published author, speaker and President Emeritus of The American Chiropractor magazine. Dr. Busch is a doctor who did not just dream about better outcomes for his patients, but a doctor who took action and made a difference.

Dr. Busch resides in Fort Wayne Indiana area with his wife Jennifer and two children.

**To contact Dr. Richard E. Busch III, write:**

> \* Surgery not Included
> C/O Dr. Richard E. Busch
> 5005 Riviera Court
> Fort Wayne, Indiana 46825

**Or visit his website at:**

> *www.surgerynotincluded.com*